Global Landscape of Nutrition Challenges in Infants and Children

Nestlé Nutrition Institute Workshop Series

Vol. 93

Global Landscape of Nutrition Challenges in Infants and Children

Editors

Kim F. Michaelsen Copenhagen
Lynnette M. Neufeld Geneva
Andrew M. Prentice Banjul

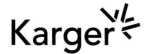

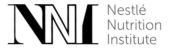

© 2020 Nestlé Nutrition Institute, Switzerland
CH 1814 La Tour-de-Peilz
S. Karger AG, P.O. Box, CH–4009 Basel (Switzerland) www.karger.com

Library of Congress Cataloging-in-Publication Data

Names: Nestlé Nutrition Workshop (93rd : 2019 : Kolkata, India), author. |
  Michaelsen, Kim Fleischer, editor. | Neufeld, Lynnette M., editor. |
  Prentice, Andrew, editor. | Nestlé Nutrition Institute, issuing body.
Title: Global landscape of nutrition challenges in infants and children /
  editors, Kim F. Michaelsen, Lynnette M. Neufeld, Andrew M. Prentice.
Other titles: Nestlé Nutrition Institute workshop series ; v. 93.
  1664-2147
Description: Basel ; New York : Karger ; Switzerland : Nestlé Nutrition
  Institute, [2020] | Series: Nestlé Nutrition Institute workshop series,
  1664-2147 ; vol. 93 | Includes bibliographical references and index. |
  Summary: "This book covers learning from the 93rd Nestle Nutrition
  Institute Workshop Series held in March 2019, which focused on infants
  and children, specifically the importance of nutrition both prior to
  conception and in children beyond two years of age. Three sessions
  covered an updated picture of global malnutrition, the role of milk in
  early life, and the ramifications of environmental constraints to
  healthy child growth. Taken together, the three sessions provide an
  update and overview of diverse issues relevant to the epidemiology and
  biology of nutrition in early life, programmatic implications, and
  future directions"-- Provided by publisher.
Identifiers: LCCN 2019058457 (print) | LCCN 2019058458 (ebook) | ISBN
  9783318066487 (hardcover ; alk. paper) | ISBN 9783318066494 (ebook)
Subjects: MESH: Child Nutritional Physiological Phenomena | Global Health |
  Child | Infant | Congress
Classification: LCC RJ206 (print) | LCC RJ206 (ebook) | NLM W1 NE228D
  v.93 2020 | DDC 362.19892--dc23
LC record available at https://lccn.loc.gov/2019058457
LC ebook record available at https://lccn.loc.gov/2019058458

Printed on acid-free and non-aging paper (ISO 9706)
ISBN 978–3–318–06648–7
e-ISBN 978–3–318–06649–4
ISSN 1664–2147
e-ISSN 1664–2155

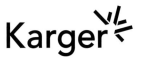

Basel · Freiburg · Paris · London · New York · Chennai · New Delhi ·
Bangkok · Beijing · Shanghai · Tokyo · Kuala Lumpur · Singapore · Sydney

Contents

VII **Preface**

IX **Foreword**

XI **Contributors**

Pediatric Nutrition: Challenges and Approaches to Address Them

1 **Global Landscape of Malnutrition in Infants and Young Children**
Neufeld, L.M.; Beal, T. (Switzerland); Larson, L.M. (Australia);
Cattaneo, F.D. (Switzerland)

15 **When Does It All Begin: What, When, and How Young Children Are Fed**
Bentley, M.E.; Nulty, A.K. (USA)

25 **Improving Children's Diet: Approach and Progress**
Ramakrishnan, U.; Webb Girard, A. (USA)

39 **The Importance of Food Composition Data for Estimating
Micronutrient Intake: What Do We Know Now and into the Future?**
Grande, F. (Brazil); Vincent, A. (Australia)

51 **Balancing Safety and Potential for Impact in Universal Iron
Interventions**
Baldi, A.J.; Larson, L.M.; Pasricha, S.-R. (Australia)

63 **Summary on Pediatric Nutrition: Challenges and Approaches to Address
Them**
Neufeld, L.M. (Switzerland)

Role of Milk in Early Life

67 **Human Milk as the First Source of Micronutrients**
Allen, L.H.; Hampel, D. (USA)

77 **Role of Milk and Dairy Products in Growth of the Child**
Grenov, B.; Larnkjær, A.; Mølgaard, C.; Michaelsen, K.F. (Denmark)

91 **Vitamin B12: An Intergenerational Story**
Chittaranjan, Y. (India)

103 **Vegan Diet in Young Children**
Müller, P. (Switzerland)

111 **Role of Optimized Plant Protein Combinations as a Low-Cost Alternative to Dairy Ingredients in Foods for Prevention and Treatment of Moderate Acute Malnutrition and Severe Acute Malnutrition**
Manary, M.; Callaghan-Gillespie, M. (USA)

121 **Summary on the Role of Milk in Early Life**
Michaelsen, K.F. (Denmark)

Environmental Impacts on Nutrition

125 **Environmental and Physiological Barriers to Child Growth and Development**
Prentice, A.M. (The Gambia)

133 **The Gut Microbiome in Child Malnutrition**
Robertson, R.C. (UK)

145 **Intergenerational Influences on Child Development: An Epigenetic Perspective**
Silver, M.J. (UK)

153 **Summarizing the Child Growth and Diarrhea Findings of the Water, Sanitation, and Hygiene Benefits and Sanitation Hygiene Infant Nutrition Efficacy Trials**
Makasi, R.R. (Zimbabwe); Humphrey, J.H. (Zimbabwe/USA)

167 **Summary of Environmental Impacts on Nutrition**
Prentice, A.M. (The Gambia)

173 **Subject Index**

For more information on related publications, please consult the NNI website: www.nestlenutrition-institute.org

Preface

Previous Nestlé Nutrition Institute (NNI) Workshops have covered the role of nutrition in health and disease at all stages of the life cycle. Proceedings and web-casts of all these workshops are freely available via the NNI website at www.nestlenutrition-institute.org.

Unsurprisingly, there has been a particular emphasis on the nutrition of mothers and young children with the "First 1,000 days" since this is a crucial period of early development that lays the foundation for a child's lifelong health. Relating to this period, recent workshops have focused on human milk (NNIW90), on complementary feeding (NNIW87), on protein in neonatal and infant nutrition (NNIW86), and on the low-birth weight baby – "Born too soon or too small" (NNIW81).

This 93rd workshop in the series sought to open the aperture around the first 1,000 days and considered the importance of nutrition both prior to conception and in children beyond 2 years of age. The phrase "Global Landscape" in the title was intended to capture the 2 possible meanings of global; the geographical meaning and the "holistic" meaning in which the program covered diverse as-pects of the nutritional landscape as well as the nonnutritional environmental challenges faced by so many mothers and children.

Session I provides an updated picture of malnutrition around the world, the recent progress that has been made in eliminating malnutrition in all its forms and several data limitations to track such progress. It focuses on the residual challenges facing governments and civil society as we seek to eliminate poverty-associated malnutrition, without escalating the rates of obesity. Patterns of how and what children eat as they pass through their early life stages are described, as well as the challenges of improving children's diets in settings worldwide and against the limitations imposed by poverty and by parents' poor knowledge of the principles of nutrition. The importance of accurate and comprehensive food composition data to enable reliable estimates of nutrient intakes is also covered with a strong emphasis on future methodological advances and the unique challenges of micronutrients. The final chapter provides a case study on how we balance the risks and benefits of micronutrient interventions with a special focus on the most challenging of nutrients – iron – that has huge benefits but possible risks in terms of promoting infections.

Session II covers different aspects of the role of milk in early life. New worldwide research on the determinants and content of micronutrients in human milk is described. The following chapters cover different aspects of cow's milk with a chapter on how it influences growth with a focus on linear growth. Cow's milk is an important source of vitamin B12, and the consequences and recommendations regarding a vegan diet without milk are presented. Low vitamin B12 levels are found in diets of many rural Indian populations and the effects through the life course was the next chapter. The session closes with a chapter on the possible role of optimized plant proteins as an alternative to dairy ingredients in treating children with severe acute malnutrition.

Session III widens the aperture still further by considering the ramifications of environmental constraints to healthy child growth. The chapters cover the issue of how persistent gut damage and systemic inflammation can precipitate malnutrition as well as the putative effects of alterations in the gut microbiota. There has, for many years, been great interest in the possibility that growth and health in one generation might be influenced by the health of our forebears in previous generations. This question is covered from an epigenetic perspective that examines how epigenetic mechanisms mediate intergenerational effects and might possibly mediate longer-term transgenerational effects, though the evidence for the latter is mostly lacking in humans. The final chapter covers the recent findings from the very large WASH Benefits and Shine trials in Kenya, Bangladesh, and Zimbabwe and how the research and policy agenda is evolving to support much more intense "Transformative WASH" programs.

Together the 3 sessions provide an update and overview of diverse issues relevant to the epidemiology, biology of nutrition in early life, programmatic implications, and future directions.

Kim F. Michaelsen, Copenhagen
Lynnette M. Neufeld, Geneva
Andrew M. Prentice, Banjul

Foreword

Malnutrition among children remains a persistent problem around the world. The latest UNICEF data report that nearly half of all deaths in children under 5 years of age can be attributed to undernutrition. Poor linear growth, or stunting, affects over 150 million children around the world, one-third of whom live in India. Among the 50 million children who are wasted, half are in South Asia; yet this region is also home to a large proportion of the 40 million children who are overweight.

These disquieting results raise several questions. Despite international guidelines on early childhood feeding, why does this problem persist? There is already an extensive body of literature from studies that have tested different combinations of interventions, including dietary, behavioral, educational, and social components. Although the results from these trials can be not convincing, one thing is clear: addressing any factor (or a limited number of factors) in isolation is not enough.

The aim of the 93rd Nestlé Nutrition Institute Workshop, which took place in India in March 29th–31st, 2019, was to map the challenges within the global landscape of childhood nutrition. The opening session led by Prof. Lynnette M. Neufeld outlined the key barriers faced in pediatric nutrition, from both the global and the local perspectives. Understanding the specific nutrition deficits of a particular population is a first step in addressing the problem. In addition, we must also understand local feeding practices, in order to identify suitable interventions that can strike a balance between effectiveness and safety. The second session chaired by Prof. Kim F. Michaelsen focused on the importance of milk in child growth and its role at different developmental stages during childhood. It also called attention to the key points to be aware of when feeding children a vegan diet and how to use plan protein combinations as a cost-effective alternative to cow's milk proteins for the prevention and treatment of acute malnutrition.

The final session designed by Prof. Andrew M. Prentice took a step broader in order to identify the environmental influences of nutrition. Infections from unhygienic surroundings combined with intergenerational nutritional deficits are major forces that can shape the epigenome and the infant gut microbiome. Together, these aspects of the global landscape of nutrition provide a roadmap toward combating nutritional deficiencies in vulnerable pediatric population around the world.

On behalf of the Nestle Nutrition Institute, I would like to thank the 3 Chairs of the workshop Lynnette M. Neufeld, Kim F. Michaelsen, and Andrew M. Prentice for putting the scientific program together.

We also would like to thank all speakers and scientific experts in the audience, who have contributed to the workshop content and scientific discussions.

Dr. Natalia Wagemans, MD
Global Head
Nestle Nutrition Institute, Switzerland

Contributors

Chairpersons & Speakers

Prof. Lindsay H. Allen, PhD
USDA ARS Western Human Nutrition
Research Center
430 W. Health Sciences Drive
Davis, CA 95616-5270
USA
E-Mail lindsay.allen@ars.usda.gov

Dr. Margaret E. Bentley, PhD
Health & Infectious Diseases
130 Rosenau, CB 7400
UNC Gillings School of Global Public
Health
University of North Carolina
Chapel Hill, NC 27516
USA
E-Mail pbentley@unc.edu

Dr. Fernanda Grande, PhD
Food and Agriculture Organization of
the United Nations (FAO)
108 Almeida Torres St.
Sao Paulo-SP, 01530-010
Brazil
E-Mail fernandagrande@usp.br

Prof. Jean H. Humphrey, SCD
John Hopkins Bloomberg School of
Public Health
Wolfe St. Building 2041
615 N Wolfe Street
Baltimore, MD 21205
USA
E-Mail jhumphr2@jhu.edu

Mark Manary, MD
Department of Pediatrics
St. Louis Children's Hospital
One Children's Place
St. Louis, MO 63110
USA
E-Mail manary@kids.wustl.edu

Prof. Kim F. Michaelsen
University of Copenhagen
Department of Nutrition, Exercise and
Sports
Paediatric and International Nutrition
Rolighedsvej 26
DK-1958 Frederiksberg C
Denmark
E-Mail kfm@nexs.ku.dk

Dr. Med. Pascal Müller
Children's Hospital of
Eastern Switzerland
Claudiusstrasse 6
CH-9006 St. Gallen
Switzerland
E-Mail pascal.mueller@kispisg.ch

Prof. Lynnette M. Neufeld
Director, Knowledge Leadership, Global
Alliance for Improved Nutrition (GAIN)
Rue Varembé 7
CH-1202 Geneva
Switzerland
E-Mail lneufeld@gainhealth.org

Dr. Sant-Rayn Pasricha
The Walter and Eliza Hall Institute of
Medical Research
1G Royal Parade
Parkville 3052
Australia
E-Mail pasricha.s@wehi.edu.au

Prof. Andrew M. Prentice
Head of Nutrition Theme
MRC Unit The Gambia at London
School of Hygiene & Tropical
Medicine
Atlantic Boulevard, Fajara
PO Box 273, Banjul
The Gambia
E-Mail aprentice@mrc.gm

Prof. Usha Ramakrishnan
Rollins School of Public Health
Emory University
1518 Clifton Road NE Room 7009
(404) 727-1092
Atlanta, GA 30322
USA
E-Mail uramakr@sph.emory.edu

Dr. Ruairi C. Robertson
Centre for Genomics and Child Health
Blizard Institute
Queen Mary University of London
4 Newark Street, Whitechapel
London E1 2AT
UK
E-Mail r.robertson@qmul.ac.uk

Dr. Matt J. Silver, PhD
Nutrition Theme
MRC Unit The Gambia at the London
School of Hygiene & Tropical Medicine
Keppel Street
London WC1E 7HT
UK
E-Mail Matt.Silver@lshtm.ac.uk

Prof. Chittaranjan S. Yajnik
Head of Department Diabetes Unit
KEM Hospital Research Centre, Pune
6th Floor, Banoo Coyaji Building
King Edward Memorial Hospital
Rasta Peth, Pune, 411011
Maharashtra
India
E-Mail diabetes@kemdiabetes.org

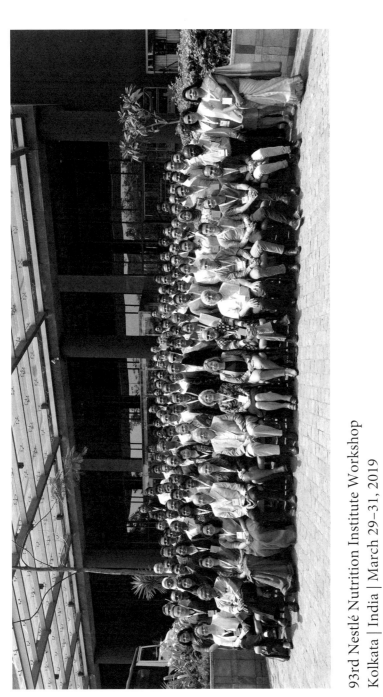

93rd Nestlé Nutrition Institute Workshop
Kolkata | India | March 29–31, 2019

Michaelsen KF, Neufeld LM, Prentice AM (eds): Global Landscape of Nutrition Challenges in
Infants and Children. Nestlé Nutr Inst Workshop Ser, vol 93, pp 1–13, (DOI: 10.1159/000503315)
Nestlé Nutrition Institute, Switzerland/S. Karger AG., Basel, © 2020

Global Landscape of Malnutrition in Infants and Young Children

Lynnette M. Neufeld[a] · Ty Beal[a] · Leila M. Larson[b] ·
Françoise D. Cattaneo[a]

[a]Global Alliance for Improved Nutrition (GAIN), Geneva, Switzerland; [b]Department of Medicine,
The University of Melbourne, Melbourne, VIC, Australia

Abstract

Malnutrition during the first years of life has immediate adverse health consequences, including increased mortality risk, and impaired long-term health and capacities. Undernutrition is an important contributor to poor linear growth, stunting, which affects over 149 million children <5 years of age worldwide, one-third of whom live in India. Over 49 million
children are wasted; yet globally, there are also 40 million overweight children. Up-to-date
data on the magnitude and distribution of micronutrient malnutrition globally and in many
countries are lacking. Anemia has been used as a proxy for micronutrient malnutrition; yet
anemia, like stunting, has a complex etiology and numerous nonnutritional as well as nutritional causes. Undernutrition, specifically stunting, wasting, and micronutrient deficiency
increasingly coexist with overweight, but accurate data to assess the extent to which these
co-exist in countries, households, and individuals and the factors that predict it are scarce.
Recent analyses in several countries suggest that there is substantial variability within and
among regions in the prevalence and determinants of malnutrition. More and better data
that can be used to tailor policies and programs to local contexts are urgently needed if we
are to accelerate progress toward addressing malnutrition in all its forms.

© 2020 Nestlé Nutrition Institute, Switzerland/S. Karger AG, Basel

The Burden of Malnutrition in All Its Forms

The term malnutrition is often used synonymously with undernutrition. During childhood, undernutrition may result in inadequate linear growth (low height-for-age or stunting) or in insufficient accumulation of body mass (low weight-for-height or wasting) [1]. Micronutrient deficiency diagnosed through clinical symptoms or biomarkers of micronutrient status below established cutoffs is an additional form of undernutrition that affects children and adults alike. It is recognized, however, that overweight and obesity and the associated noncommunicable diseases are also forms of malnutrition affecting all age groups. Global goals now seek to address malnutrition in all its forms [2]. For example, the World Health Assembly has called for a 40% reduction in the number of children who are stunted, wasting no higher than 5%, and no increase in the number of overweight children by 2025 [3].

Malnutrition during the first years of life has immediate adverse health consequences and impairs long-term health and capacities. Children who become undernourished in early life are at a higher risk of dying, are more susceptible to illness, and may suffer growth and developmental delays [4]. Infections impair growth and nutrient absorption through a variety of mechanisms, such as reduced appetite, direct nutrient losses, and increased metabolic requirements or catabolic losses of nutrients through defecation, and may weaken transport of nutrients to tissues [5]. Children with adequate nutrition during early childhood have been shown to earn 21% more in wages as adults than children who were malnourished [6]. Overweight and obesity now contribute up to 7.1% of deaths [7], and there is a growing body of evidence that the risk of overweight and obesity starts in early life and increases during adolescence and adulthood [8].

UNICEF recently published updated statistics compiling data on nutritional status of children <5 years of age from all countries with available data [9]. From 2000 to 2018, the global prevalence of stunting in children <5 years of age decreased from 32.5 to 21.9% with prevalence decreasing across all regions globally. However, stunting still affected approximately 149 million children <5 years of age in 2018. At the same time, 49.5 million children (7.3%) were wasted, and an additional 40.1 million (5.9%) were overweight. South Asia has the highest prevalence of stunting (34.4%) and wasting (15.2%). While the actual number of children affected is lower in sub-Saharan Africa given population size, stunting prevalence remains very high (≥30%) across most countries. The number of children affected by stunting is decreasing across most regions, but there was a 29% increase in West and Central Africa, due to population growth. Overweight and obesity among children are increasing globally, but with substantial variability by region. For example, in Eastern Europe and Central Asia, overweight in children increased from 8.2% in 2000 to 14.9% in 2018. In the same period, the prevalence decreased in West and Central Africa from 4.2% in 2000 to 2.8% in 2018.

Unlike anthropometric measures of malnutrition, the global burden and trends in micronutrient deficiency in children are not well quantified. For years, the figure of 2 billion people affected by micronutrient deficiency has been quoted (see for example 10). Unfortunately, the empirical evidence that underpins this estimate is weak, likely based on anemia, iodine, and vitamin A deficiency prevalence from the early 1990 [11]. Thus, it is not useful for tracking progress. Given changes in dietary patterns [12], food fortification [13], and other interventions, its appropriateness even for advocacy purposes 20+ years on is questionable.

More recent data provide national, regional, and global estimates [14]. These have been incorporated in high-quality data visualization tools [10], but data limitations persist. First, the use of anemia as a proxy for micronutrient deficiency may not be appropriate in all regions given its complex etiology (discussed further below). Second, for some nutrients there are considerable limitations to existing biomarkers of status (e.g., blood or urine levels). In the case of zinc, for example, national food balance sheets have been used to estimate the proportion of the population with inadequate intakes as a proxy for deficiency [15]. There are several limitations to this approach including the very low quality of national food balance sheets to represent actual food intake of individuals [16]. Finally, infection and inflammation affect many biomarkers of nutritional status, and until recently, there has been little consensus on how to adjust prevalence estimates to account for this. For example, in one study in Indonesia, the prevalence of iron deficiency was substantially underestimated, while vitamin A and zinc prevalence were overestimated without adjustment for inflammation [17]. The recent Biomarkers Reflecting Inflammation and Nutritional Determinants of Anemia project has now published adjustment factors for several micronutrients that should help overcome this challenge [18].

Where high-quality recent data do exist, there is substantial evidence of a high burden of micronutrient malnutrition among children. A recent review identified 14 countries with vitamin A deficiency data in children collected after 2010 and an additional 13 countries with data from 2006 to 2010, 7 from 2001 to 2005, 16 before 2000, and 32 with no nationally representative data [19]. Of the 50 countries with data, only 7 reported mild deficiency and 2 no deficiency (Guatemala, Indonesia); all others had a prevalence considered to be a moderate or severe level of vitamin A deficiency among children. Unfortunately, discrepancies between reviews of survey data where data quality can be verified and global tracking mechanisms have not been resolved. For example, the most recent national survey in Kenya (cited by Wirth et al. [19]) reported a prevalence of 9.2% (mild deficiency), compared to 84.4% (severe deficiency) reported through global tracking data [10].

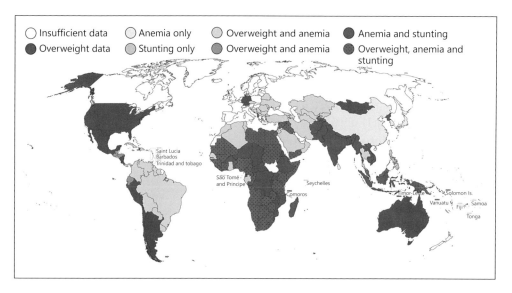

Legend (map):
- ○ Insufficient data
- ● Overweight data
- ○ Anemia only
- ○ Stunting only
- ○ Overweight and anemia
- ○ Overweight and anemia
- ● Anemia and stunting
- ◐ Overweight, anemia and stunting

Map labels: Saint Lucia, Barbados, Trinidad and tobago, São Tomé and Principe, Comoros, Seychelles, Timor-Leste, Solomon Is., Vanuatu, Fiji, Samoa, Tonga

Fig. 1. Coexistence of childhood stunting and anemia and overweight in adult women, 2017, reproduced from [7].

Other nutrients with evidence of high deficiency prevalence in children in low- and middle-income countries include iron, zinc, and iodine [20]. While data are scarce, vitamin D deficiency is likely also high among children in several countries [21]. There is also evidence that intake of essential micronutrients, specifically vitamins A, D, E and calcium, is insufficient among many children in high-income countries [22]. There is an urgent need for greater investment in the collection and use of high-quality survey data to quantify the magnitude and distribution of micronutrient malnutrition and ensure that programmatic responses are appropriately targeted.

There is growing evidence that many countries are affected by both undernutrition (stunting, wasting, micronutrient malnutrition) and overweight/obesity, often referred to as the double burden of malnutrition. For example, the 2018 Global Nutrition Report [7] mapped the coexistence of stunting in children <5 years of age and anemia and overweight in adult women (Fig. 1). This pattern has important policy implications as countries must deal with undernutrition simultaneously with overweight, obesity, and related noncommunicable diseases. Such national-level data, however, provide no indication whether the issues are concentrated in the same subsets of the population (e.g., geographical regions, urban vs. rural areas), the same households (e.g., overweight mother and undernourished child), or whether the same individuals are affected by >1 forms of malnutrition (e.g., stunted, overweight, micronutrient-deficient child). Much survey data exist that, if analyzed, would allow for more comprehensive estimates of the co-existence of nutritional issues in population subgroups, households, and individuals to inform policy and programs. There is also a need for more comparable approaches to quantifying and studying the determinants of the double burden of malnutrition among countries to permit global tracking [23].

Progress Toward Addressing Malnutrition: Some Examples from the Literature

Several countries have made substantial progress addressing malnutrition in children. In Nepal, for example, stunting declined from 57.1% (2000) to 36.0% (2017), and in Lesotho from 52.7 to 33.4% over the same period [24]. In Brazil, stunting declined from 19% in 1990 to 7% by 2006 [2]. Several of the likely determinants to progress in Brazil include significant increase in exclusive breastfeeding prevalence (2% in the 1980 to 39% in 2006), and important reductions in open defecation (17% in 1990 to 2% in 2011) and in extreme poverty, with the proportion of the population living on <2 USD per day dropping from 21 to 5% over the same period [2]. Despite these promising cases, many countries are not on track to reach global targets of stunting and wasting reduction and no increase in overweight [7]. Unfortunately, well over 100 countries have no data to adequately track such targets [7].

Even where data exist, tracking national progress often masks substantial disparity of malnutrition in children within countries. A recent publication from India illustrates this issue dramatically. Using stunting prevalence data by district from a 2015 to 2016 survey, the authors illustrate the dramatic variation in stunting prevalence across India (Fig. 2) [25]. The variation between districts with the highest (>40%) and lowest (<20%) rates of stunting was explained by several maternal factors (low BMI, marriage <18 years of age, antenatal care), adequacy of the child diet, several demographic and economic factors (10+ years of schooling, household size, and assets), while 29% of the variation remained unexplained. This has important implications for policy and programmatic responses that must consider the severity of the issues and the diversity across regions of the underlying determinants.

While many countries lack data to assess variability of prevalence disaggregated to this level, several factors that strongly predict disparity in the prevalence of malnutrition are well documented. For example, globally and in all regions, children living in the poorest households are at least twice as likely to be stunted than the richest [9]. In Latin America and the Caribbean, the prevalence of stunting among poor families (30%) is 4.3 times higher than that among the richest (7%). Similar analyses to explore the prevalence of overweight in children among diverse population subgroups within countries have not yet been

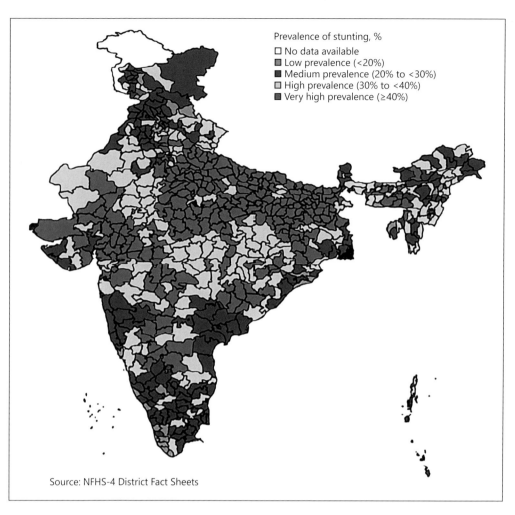

Prevalence of stunting, %
☐ No data available
■ Low prevalence (<20%)
■ Medium prevalence (20% to <30%)
☐ High prevalence (30% to <40%)
■ Very high prevalence (≥40%)

Source: NFHS-4 District Fact Sheets

Fig. 2. Diversity in the prevalence of childhood stunting by district in India, using data from 2015 to 2016, reproduced from [25]. NFHS, National Family Health Survey.

compiled at global level. Several publications suggest, however, that overweight among children, while once concentrated among the non-poor, may no longer track economic boundaries as stunting does (see for example [26]).

Understanding the Etiology of Malnutrition

The determinants of undernutrition are well documented and have been recently updated to incorporate all forms of malnutrition [2]. Immediate causes include health-related behaviors (e.g., diet, activity, hygiene) and biological factors (e.g.,

Neufeld · Beal · Larson · Cattaneo

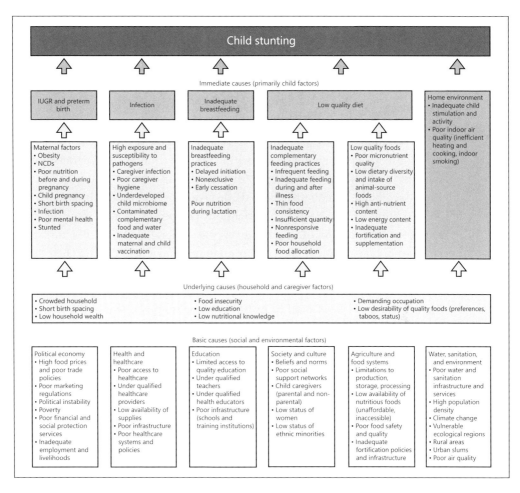

Fig. 3. Conceptual framework on the determinants of child growth. Developed by the authors building on previously published frameworks [27, 28]. IUGR, Intra-uterine growth retardation; NCDs, Non-communicable diseases.

disease state, genetics). Underlying these are several household- and community-level factors that facilitate or limit a household's ability to provide health, care, and a quality diet, such as access to food and health care, social norms related to care and feeding, and the living environment (e.g., built spaces and water and sanitation services). These factors are in turn affected by income and inequality, trade, urbanization, existence of social protection and health systems, and agricultural development, among other factors. Finally, the extent to which such factors may favor nutrition depends on an enabling environment of political commitment, effective governance, and capacity. As illustrated above in the case of Brazil, progress to address malnutrition has typically been better when policies and programs address such determinants simultaneously, accompanied by economic growth [2].

Stunting

Building on prior frameworks [27, 28], Figure 3 shows known determinants of child stunting organized along a simplified pathway. Being born small, unimproved sanitation, and diarrhea are important risk factors for stunting globally and particularly in South Asia [29]. Low maternal height and household wealth are also important predictors in South Asia [30]. The relationships between stunting and its determinants as well as their relative importance can vary substantially by context, even within a single country, as illustrated previously in India [27]. Within-country diversity in the drivers of stunting has also been documented in Vietnam [28]. Effective action to accelerate progress to address stunting may require interventions tailored to address these determinants, the composition of which may vary by geography or other factors. Path analyses of linear growth faltering using longitudinal data can also help identify where and how to intervene across the range of basic to immediate causes of stunting [31]. While data may be limiting in some contexts, in others, existing data have not been used to its full potential to document and understand the many determinants of child malnutrition and their variability by geographic or other factors like those from India and Vietnam. Longitudinal datasets are particularly powerful for understanding determinants but are rare and usually do not have sufficient geographically representation to explore variability within countries.

Anemia

As noted above, anemia continues to be the only indicator tracked consistently at a national level and used as a proxy for micronutrient status, and it is often interpreted as synonymous with iron deficiency. The determinants of anemia, however, include a complex pattern of biological, infectious, environmental, and genetic factors [32]. Anemia may be related to inadequate intakes of iron, folic acid, vitamin A, and/or vitamin B12. Conditions that cause increased loss or reduced absorption or utilization of iron such as soil-transmitted helminths, malaria, schistosomiasis, and other parasitic infections may also result in anemia, even if intakes appear adequate. Finally, genetic disorders that affect iron or hemoglobin metabolism also result in anemia.

Particularly in low- and middle-income countries, several risk factors may simultaneously cause anemia in an individual. For instance, in sub-Saharan Africa, malaria and iron deficiency are both highly prevalent. In these cases, common approaches to prevent and treat anemia, such as iron supplementation, may not be effective, and recent evidence suggests that iron supplementation may even exacerbate infection. In a study of children living in malaria-endemic Tanzania, prophylactic iron supplementation in-

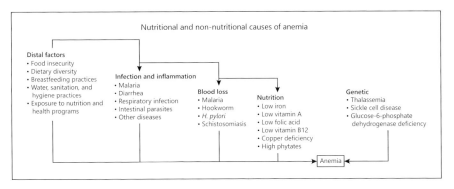

Fig. 4. Schematic illustration of the nutritional and nonnutritional causes of anemia in children and women. Developed by the authors based on results of a path analysis of anemia determinants in Uttar Pradesh, India [38].

creased the risk of hospitalization, death, malaria, and other infections among those who were not iron deficient [33]. Consumption of iron-containing multiple micronutrient powders also resulted in increased diarrhea in a study in Pakistan [34] and increased hospitalizations in Ghana [35]. Thus, understanding the etiology of anemia and a balanced assessment of the potential risks and benefits of iron supplementation should be a part of program planning [36].

In India, the prevalence of anemia is very high with little progress made over the past decade [37]; a better understanding of the etiology of anemia in context could help inform more appropriate approaches to its reduction. A recent study in Uttar Pradesh, India, examined the etiology of anemia in women and children using a state-representative survey [38]. This comprehensive study measured a range of genetic, environmental, infectious, and nutritional risk factors for anemia (Fig. 4). Results indicate that iron was an important contributor to anemia; 78% of children and 74% of women with anemia had iron deficiency anemia. Other direct and indirect determinants included inflammation, folic acid, vitamin B12, and vitamin A (serum retinol), as well as more distal factors, such as dietary diversity, household hunger, and water, sanitation, and hygiene, which work through effects on status indicators. In this population without malaria (<1%) and minimum intestinal parasites (<9%), iron and inflammation were strong determinants of hemoglobin concentration and anemia. The relationship between iron and inflammation, however, is not straightforward, and the extent to which iron and other nutritional interventions can be fully effective to address anemia is not clear. Nonnutritional causes of anemia may inhibit a response to iron interventions if not concurrently addressed. The type of analysis conducted with

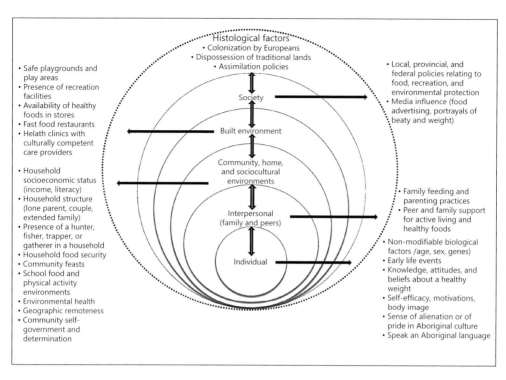

Fig. 5. The ecological model applied to determinants of obesity in children living in First Nations communities in Canada, reproduced with permission from [41].

the data from Uttar Pradesh should be used to guide effective programs in populations where the contribution of nutritional and nonnutritional determinants to anemia prevalence may vary, such as settings with malaria or high proportions of genetic abnormalities.

Overweight

There is still much to learn about the determinants and potential actions to prevent and control childhood overweight. As with stunting and anemia, the etiology of excess weight in childhood is complex and includes interactions among genetic makeup, intrauterine factors, the home and built environment, and behavioral factors [39, 40]. The interrelationship among these factors and how they may influence child weight is nicely illustrated for First Nations communities in Canada [41]. In this context, historical factors and persistent inequities dramatically influence many social and environmental determinants of overweight. An ecological model that frames biological and interpersonal determinants in this context, as illustrated in Figure 5, is helpful for identifying opportunities for action as well as potential barriers to their effectiveness. To date, few low- and middle-income countries have such in-depth analyses of the determinants of overweight in children needed to inform comprehensive approaches to addressing it.

Conclusion

Through the Sustainable Development Goals, the world has set the ambitious aim to achieve food security and end malnutrition in all its forms by 2030 [42]. Progress to achieving this goal for children is lagging, and the global prevalence of stunting, wasting, overweight, and micronutrient malnutrition remains unacceptably high. Several countries have made progress to address stunting, but many are unlikely to achieve the targets unless progress is accelerated substantially [7]. Childhood overweight is increasing in most regions, and with the limited data available, little progress has been made to addressing micronutrient malnutrition. Equally concerning is the lack of up-to-date representative data of the magnitude and distribution of malnutrition in all its forms and their determinants at national and subnational level. Beyond simply tracking progress, a more profound understanding of the contextual etiology of the various forms of malnutrition is urgently needed to inform effective action.

Disclosure Statement

The authors have no conflicts of interest to declare.

References

1 Williams AM, Suchdev PS: Assessing and improving childhood nutrition and growth globally. Pediatr Clin North Am 2017;64:755–768.
2 International Food Policy Research Institute. Global Nutrition Report: From Promise to Impact: Ending Malnutrition by 2030. Washington DC, 2016.
3 WHO. Global nutrition targets 2025: stunting policy brief (WHO/NMH/NHD/14.3). Geneva: World Health Organization; 2014.
4 Black MM, Walker SP, Fernald LC, et al: Early childhood development coming of age: Science through the life course. Lancet 2017;389:77–90.
5 Stephensen CB: Burden of infection on growth failure. J Nutr 1999;129(2S suppl):534S–538S.
6 Hoddinott J, Behrman JR, Maluccio JA, et al: Adult consequences of growth failure in early childhood. Am J Clin Nutr 2013;98:1170–1178.
7 Fanzo J, Hawkes C: 2018 Global Nutrition Report. Dev Initiat 2018 (cited March 19, 2019). https://globalnutritionreport.org/reports/global-nutrition-report-2018/.
8 John CC, Black MM, Nelson CA 3rd: Neurodevelopment: the impact of nutrition and inflammation during early to middle childhood in low-resource settings. Pediatrics 2017;139(suppl 1):S59–S71.
9 UNICEF: Malnutrition in Children. UNICEF DATA 2018 (cited March 19, 2019). https://data.unicef.org/topic/nutrition/malnutrition/.

10 Ritchie H, Roser M: Micronutrient Deficiency. Our World Data 2017 (cited April 11, 2019). https://ourworldindata.org/micronutrient-deficiency.

11 FAO: Preventing Micronutrient Malnutrition a Guide to Food-Based Approaches – Why Policy Makers Should Give Priority to Food-Based Strategies. Food and Agriculture Organization of the United Nations (cited May 14, 2019). http://www.fao.org/3/x0245e/x0245e01.htm#P38_2721.

12 Popkin BM, Gordon-Larsen P: The nutrition transition: worldwide obesity dynamics and their determinants. Int J Obes Relat Metab Disord 2004;28(suppl 3):S2–S9.

13 Osendarp SJ, Martinez H, Garrett GS, et al: Large-scale food fortification and biofortification in low- and middle-income countries: a review of programs, trends, challenges, and evidence gaps. Food Nutr Bull 2018;39:315–331.

14 World Health Organization: Vitamin and Mineral Nutrition Information System (VMNIS)|Micronutrients database (cited May 14, 2019). Geneva, Switzerland, WHO. http://www.who.int/vmnis/database/en/.

15 Wessells KR, Brown KH: Estimating the global prevalence of zinc deficiency: results based on zinc availability in national food supplies and the prevalence of stunting. PLoS One 2012;7:e50568.

16 Beal T, Massiot E, Arsenault JE, et al: Global trends in dietary micronutrient supplies and estimated prevalence of inadequate intakes. PLoS One 2017;12:e0175554.

17 Diana A, Haszard JJ, Purnamasari DM, et al: Iron, zinc, vitamin A and selenium status in a cohort of Indonesian infants after adjusting for inflammation using several different approaches. Br J Nutr 2017;118:830–839.

18 Stoltzfus RJ, Klemm R: Research, policy, and programmatic considerations from the biomarkers reflecting inflammation and nutritional determinants of anemia (BRINDA) project. Am J Clin Nutr 2017;106(suppl 1):428S–434S.

19 Wirth JP, Petry N, Tanumihardjo SA, et al: Vitamin A supplementation programs and country-level evidence of vitamin A deficiency. Nutrients 2017;9:pii:E190.

20 Harika R, Faber M, Samuel F, et al: Are low intakes and deficiencies in iron, vitamin A, zinc, and iodine of public health concern in Ethiopian, Kenyan, Nigerian, and South African children and adolescents? Food Nutr Bull 2017;38:405–427.

21 Roth DE, Abrams SA, Aloia J, et al: Global prevalence and disease burden of vitamin D deficiency: a roadmap for action in low- and middle-income countries. Ann N Y Acad Sci 2018;1430:44–79.

22 Hilger J, Goerig T, Weber P, et al: Micronutrient intake in healthy toddlers: A multinational perspective. Nutrients 2015;7:6938–6955.

23 Kosaka S, Umezaki M: A systematic review of the prevalence and predictors of the double burden of malnutrition within households. Br J Nutr 2017;117:1118–1127.

24 UNICEF, WHO, World Bank Group Joint Child Malnutrition Estimates. Levels and Trends in Child Malnutrition – Key finds of the 2018 edition. y: the Data and Analytics Section of the Division of Data, Research and Policy, UNICEF, 2018.

25 Menon P, Headey D, Avula R, et al: Understanding the geographical burden of stunting in India: a regression-decomposition analysis of district-level data from 2015–2016. Matern Child Nutr 2018;14:e12620.

26 Ranjani H, Pradeepa R, Mehreen TS, et al: Determinants, consequences and prevention of childhood overweight and obesity: an Indian context. Indian J Endocrinol Metab 2014;18(suppl 1):S17–S25.

27 Stewart CP, Iannotti L, Dewey KG, et al: Contextualising complementary feeding in a broader framework for stunting prevention. Matern Child Nutr 2013;9(suppl 2):27–45.

28 Beal T, Tumilowicz A, Sutrisna A, et al: A review of child stunting determinants in Indonesia. Matern Child Nutr 2018;14:e12617.

29 Danaei G, Andrews KG, Sudfeld CR, et al: Risk factors for childhood stunting in 137 developing countries: a comparative risk assessment analysis at global, regional, and country levels. PLoS Med 2016;13:e1002164.

30 Kim R, Mejía-Guevara I, Corsi DJ, et al: Relative importance of 13 correlates of child stunting in South Asia: insights from nationally representative data from Afghanistan, Bangladesh, India, Nepal, and Pakistan. Soc Sci Med 2017;187:144–154.

31 Prado EL, Yakes Jimenez E, Vosti S, et al: Path analyses of risk factors for linear growth faltering in four prospective cohorts of young children in Ghana, Malawi and Burkina Faso. BMJ Glob Health 2019;4:e001155.

32 Balarajan Y, Ramakrishnan U, Ozaltin E, et al: Anaemia in low-income and middle-income countries. Lancet 2011;378:2123–2135.

33 Sazawal S, Black RE, Ramsan M, et al: Effects of routine prophylactic supplementation with iron and folic acid on admission to hospital and mortality in preschool children in a high malaria transmission setting: community-based, randomised, placebo-controlled trial. Lancet 2006; 367:133–143.

34 Soofi S, Cousens S, Iqbal S, et al: Effect of provision of daily zinc and iron with several micronutrients on growth and morbidity among young children in Pakistan: a cluster-randomised trial. Lancet 2013;382:29–40.

35 Zlotkin S, Newton S, Aimone AM, et al: Effect of iron fortification on malaria incidence in infants and young children in ghana: a randomized trial. JAMA 2013;310:938–947.

36 Pasricha S: Balancing safety and potential for impact in micronutrient interventions. In: Michaelsen KF, Neufeld LM, Prentice AM (eds): Global Landscape of Nutrition Challenges in Infants and Children. Nestlé Nutr Inst Workshop Ser, vol 93, pp 51–62.

37 Nguyen PH, Scott S, Avula R, Tran LM, et al: Trends and drivers of change in the prevalence of anaemia among 1 million women and children in India, 2006 to 2016. BMJ Glob Health 2018; 3:e001010.

38 Larson LM, Thomas T, Kurpad AV, et al: Anemia in Women and Children in Uttar Pradesh, India: the Contribution of Nutritional, Environmental, Infectious, Genetic, and Underlying Social Determinants. Buenos Aires, Presentation at the 21st International Congress of Nutrition (IUNS), 2017.

39 Ang YN, Wee BS, Poh BK, et al: Multifactorial Influences of Childhood Obesity. Curr Obes Rep 2013;2:10–22.

40 Bates CR, Buscemi J, Nicholson LM, et al: Links between the organization of the family home environment and child obesity: a systematic review. Obes Rev 2018;19:716–727.

41 Willows ND, Hanley AJG, Delormier T: A socio-ecological framework to understand weight-related issues in Aboriginal children in Canada. Appl Physiol Nutr Metab 2012 37:1–13.

42 Sustainable Development Foals Fund: Goal 2: Zero hunger. Sustainable Development Goals Fund 2015 (cited April 23, 2019). http://www.sdgfund.org/goal-2-zero-hunger.

Pediatric Nutrition: Challenges and Approaches to Address Them

Michaelsen KF, Neufeld LM, Prentice AM (eds): Global Landscape of Nutrition Challenges in
Infants and Children. Nestlé Nutr Inst Workshop Ser, vol 93, pp 15–24, (DOI: 10.1159/000503353)
Nestlé Nutrition Institute, Switzerland/S. Karger AG., Basel, © 2020

When Does It All Begin: What, When, and How Young Children Are Fed

Margaret E. Bentley · Alison K. Nulty

University of North Carolina, Chapel Hill, NC, USA

Abstract

The first 2 years of life are a critical period to promote nutrition and dietary behaviors for optimal growth and development. Exclusive breastfeeding is recommended until 6 months with the addition of safe, nutritionally adequate complementary foods thereafter. Caregiver adherence to international guidelines for feeding infants and toddlers varies depending on the setting, access to information, quality of food, and cultural beliefs. Caregiver feeding style also plays an important role in what foods and drinks are offered and whether young children accept those foods. Feeding guidelines often include what is called "responsive feeding," which is the importance of caregiver attention to child cues of hunger and satiety. While there are data on food consumption and dietary diversity in early childhood, the literature on early childhood beverage consumption is limited. With the increased consumption and availability of sugar-sweetened beverages, future research should aim to understand the status of global beverage consumption among children under 2 years old and its impact on growth and development. This chapter highlights current infant and young child feeding recommendations, what young children eat and drink, and the role that parental feeding styles can have on diet and early childhood outcomes.

© 2020 Nestlé Nutrition Institute, Switzerland/S. Karger AG, Basel

Introduction

It is well established that the first 1,000 days of life are a critical period of rapid growth and development. During this period, adequate nutrition is required to meet the nutrient needs for proper growth [1]. Yet, malnutrition remains a global concern among children under 5 years of age. Malnutrition includes those who are both over- and underweight – impacting all ages. Globally, almost 240 million children under age 5 are suffering from malnutrition [2]. According to a recent World Health Organization (WHO) report, 45% of deaths in children under age 5 are due to malnutrition [3]. While many malnourished children are stunted or wasted, an increasing number are becoming overweight due to the nutrition transition [4]. The transition is causing a shift in dietary and physical activity patterns with an increase in consumption of sugars and fat and a decrease in daily physical activity. The transition was initiated by a variety of changes within the economy as well as improvements to technology [5].

This chapter provides a brief review of both global patterns and selective data from India, where the 93rd Nestlé Nutrition Institute Workshop on "Global Landscape of Nutrition Challenges in Children" occurred. It focuses on infant and young child feeding (IYCF) recommendations and global adherence, the importance of caregiver feeding style and its impact on growth and development, and how nutrition interventions and future research can be used to improve current IYCF practices.

Global Infant Young Child Feeding Recommendations
Both the WHO and the United Nations International Children's Emergency Fund (UNICEF) have published IYCF guidelines to ensure children are receiving adequate nutrition that promotes proper growth and development through childhood. The guidelines recommend that mothers initiate breastfeeding within 1 hour of birth and to breastfeed exclusively for the first 6 months of life [6]. Early initiation and exclusive breastfeeding provide multiple benefits to infants such as decreased risk of infant mortality and increased protection against disease [7]. Victora et al. conducted a review of 28 meta-analyses on the associations between breastfeeding and its corresponding maternal/child outcomes [8]. Results showed breastfed infants had a decreased risk of death, diarrhea, and respiratory infections compared to those who were not breastfed [8].

At 6 months, the WHO and UNICEF recommend introducing nutritionally adequate, safe complementary food while continuing to breastfeed. They specify to begin by introducing iron-rich foods with no specific order thereafter. In low-access settings, fortified foods or vitamin–mineral supplements may be needed [6, 9]. Complementary feeding (CF) should begin with small portions of food that gradually increase as the child develops [6]. Failure to adhere to these recommendations during early childhood has been linked to long-term growth impairment and is directly associated with an increased risk of illness [10].

The WHO also published IYCF recommendations specific to mothers living with HIV. "Mothers living with HIV should breastfeed for at least 12 months and may continue breastfeeding for up to 24 months or beyond while being fully supported for ART adherence" [11]. In special circumstances, for example, if the mother is temporarily ill and unable to breastfeed, the recommendation is to express and heat-treat the breastmilk before providing it to the infant [11]. These recommendations were informed by the results of multiple IYCF interventions and systematic reviews [11, 12].

While the WHO and UNICEF guidelines are global recommendations, some countries have their own national IYCF guidelines as well. For example, in 2015, India finalized their *Optimal and Appropriate Infant and Young Child Nutrition Practices and Strategies* after consulting with a variety of infant feeding experts such as partners from the WHO, UNICEF, Ministry of Child Welfare Department, and the Human Milk Banking Association of India [13]. Most of these guidelines align with the WHO and UNICEF recommendations, including the guideline that specifies to practice *responsive feeding* (RF). For caregivers, RF involves recognizing and encouraging a child's hunger and fullness cues and responding accordingly [14, 15]. The importance and the impact of RF are discussed further below.

Assessment of IYCF

Many early childhood nutrition interventions and programs target IYCF practices. To assess the potential effect of these interventions, the WHO has published 15 IYCF indicators [16]. Eight of the 15 are classified as core, these include early initiation of breastfeeding, exclusive breastfeeding under 6 months, continued breastfeeding for 1 year, introduction of solid, semi-solid, or soft foods, consumption of iron-rich or iron-fortified foods, minimum dietary diversity (MDD), minimum meal frequency (MMF), and minimum acceptable diet (MAD) [16]. These indicators provide the ability to evaluate and track feeding practices and patterns both within a country and globally.

Adherence to IYCF Recommendations

Breastfeeding

Early initiation of breastfeeding, within the first hour of life, provides many benefits to the newborn infant. First, it ensures the infant receives colostrum. Colostrum is important because it is rich in antibodies that confer passive immunity to the infant [7, 17]. Compared to infants who were put to breast within 1 hour of birth, the risk of death is 41% higher for those who initiated 2–23 h after birth and 79% higher for those who initiated 1 day or longer after birth [7]. Globally, only 41% of infants were put to breast within

Table 1. Child feeding practices and nutritional status of children in India comparing NFHS-4 and NFHS-3

Child feeding practices and nutritional status of children	NFHS-4 (2015–2016)	NFHS-3 (2005–2006)
Children under age 3 years breastfed within 1 h of birth, %	41.6	23.4
Children under age 6 months exclusively breastfed, %	54.9	46.4
Children age 6–8 months receiving solid or semi-solid food and breastmilk, %	42.7	52.6
Breastfeeding children age 6–23 months receiving an adequate diet, %	8.7	N/A
Non-breastfeeding children age 6–23 months receiving an adequate diet, %	14.3	N/A
Total children age 6–23 months receiving an adequate diet, %	9.6	N/A

1 hour of birth between years 2013 and 2018 [18]. East Asia and the Pacific region had the lowest rates with 32%, while the highest rates occurred in Eastern and Southern Africa at 65% [18]. In India, a nationally representative household survey conducted in 2015–2016 found that 41.6% of children under 3 years old had been breastfed within 1 hour of birth. This was a positive increase compared to the survey conducted in 2005–2006, where 23.4% of children under 3 years old had been breastfed within 1 hour of birth (Table 1) [19, 20].

In addition to the multiple benefits of early initiation, breastfeeding initiation within the first hour of life increases the likelihood of exclusive breastfeeding through the first 6 months [7]. Despite the important benefits of breastfeeding, less than half of all infants are exclusively breastfed through the first 6 months of life [18]. The most recent data from UNICEF show global exclusive breastfeeding rates at 41%. East Asia and the Pacific region had the lowest rates of exclusive breastfeeding at 22%, while Eastern and Southern Africa had the highest rates at 56% [18]. Within India, the exclusive breastfeeding rate was 54.9% in 2015–2016, compared to 46.4% in 2005–2006 (Table 1) [19, 20].

Multiple factors influence why mothers do not exclusively breastfeed, including beliefs and cultural norms [21]. Mothers encounter multiple challenges that discourage exclusive breastfeeding through 6 months of age. Prenatally, women who lack access to breastfeeding information and education are less likely to initiate after birth [22]. During labor, both the maternal labor experience and the breastfeeding attitudes of the hospital staff can impact the maternal breastfeeding intention, which is associated with early weaning [23]. In the postpartum period, women who have clinical problems, such as low supply or problems with infant latch, are more likely to discontinue breastfeeding. Women who identify a lack of clinical/provider support are more likely to discontinue breastfeeding before 6 months. Also, women who return to work before 6 months are less likely to be exclusively breastfeeding for 6 months [24–26].

Complementary Feeding

As noted above, the guidelines recommend exclusive breastfeeding until infants are 6 months of age with the gradual introduction of nutritionally safe and adequate complementary foods [6]. To measure adequacy of CF, the WHO indicators defined above are used: MDD, MMF, and MAD [16]. Dietary diversity reflects a nutritionally adequate diet. Children aged 6–23 months should eat food from at least 4 of the following food groups a day: grains, roots and tubers, legumes and nuts, dairy products, meat and fish, eggs, Vitamin A-rich fruits and vegetables, and other fruits and vegetables. A diet lacking in diversity can increase a child's risk of micronutrient deficiencies [7]. Yet, only 29% of the world's children meet the requirements [27]. Additionally, children need to eat frequently throughout the day to meet their energy and nutrient requirements. However, only 50% of young children (6–23 months) are meeting the MMF requirements. Among children under 2 years old, there is an equity gap between rich and poor for both MDD and MMF [7]. Globally, children from poorer households consume less diverse and more infrequent meals compared to those from richer households. Low maternal education levels and maternal media exposure were also associated with suboptimal CF practices in multiple countries [28–33].

Within India, the only CF indicator evaluated in both the 2005–2006 and the 2015–2016 national surveys was the percent of children aged 6–8 months receiving solid or semi-solid food and breastmilk [19, 20]. The percent of children who received solid or semi-solid food and breastmilk decreased by 10%, despite data that showed the breastfeeding indicators substantially increased during this period (Table 1) [19, 20]. While the reasons for this decrease are not clear, CF programs and policies should be strengthened as part of infant and young child nutrition (IYCN) programs.

Accompanying the nutrition transition, multinational beverage companies and their products are more accessible worldwide [34]. Global data on child beverage consumption is extremely limited, especially among children under 2 years old. Most of the literature is specific to the United States and results from the Feeding Infants and Toddlers Study [35]. From the Feeding Infants and Toddlers Study data, Kay et al. [35] found that breastmilk and formula were the top

2 beverages consumed among children younger than 12 months, and as expected, cow's milk consumption continued to increase as children aged. Children older than 12 months had an average 100% juice consumption of 8 ounces per day, almost twice the recommended amount [35, 36].

Beverage data are limited within India as well. An analysis of the 2005–2006 Indian National Family Health Survey showed that nearly 10% of children (ages 6–59 months) had not consumed any water in the last 24 h [37]. Of those children, over 50% reported not drinking any beverages, while a quarter reported drinking 2 or more beverages such as tea, coffee, or juice. Children over 2 years old were more likely to consume non-milk beverages compared to younger children. The authors found in settings where water is scarce, sugar-sweetened beverages, such as juice or soda, are more widely consumed among younger children [37]. More global data on beverage consumption during early childhood are needed to track sugar-sweetened beverage consumption and its impact on growth throughout early childhood.

Caregiver Feeding Styles

Not only do caregivers play a prominent role in what and when children are fed, they also determine *how* children are fed. Parental feeding styles play a significant role in establishing healthy behaviors for optimal growth and development [38]. The WHO recommends that parents and caregivers practice RF [14]. According to Black and Aboud RF, includes "(1) ensuring that the feeding context is pleasant with few distractions; (2) encouraging and attending to the child's signals of hunger and satiety; and (3) responding to the child in a prompt, emotionally supportive, contingent, and developmentally appropriate manner" [15]. Non-RF is defined as "A lack of reciprocity between the parent and child, with the caregiver taking excessive control of the feeding situation (pressuring or restricting food intake), the child completely controlling the feeding situation (indulgent), or the caregiver being uninvolved during meals (laissez faire)" [39]. The importance of the dyadic relationship and the role of infant temperament play a role in how caregiver feeding style may be influenced. For example, caregivers who perceive infants to be "fussy" or "active" may introduce complementary foods more often, as a way to sooth a crying or an active infant [40, 41]. Research on feeding styles and its association with breastfeeding and growth outcomes has been conducted in high-, middle-, and low-income countries [42–44]. Although researchers recognize the importance of RF, there are limited data to assess how RF messages combined with improved CF behaviors contribute to child diet or growth.

An observational study of 100 meal time observations of children aged 12–23 months in rural Ethiopia reported that caregivers of stunted children had poorer IYCF practices, such as being less responsive to the child's hunger and satiation cues, compared to caregivers of non-stunted children [45]. A randomized controlled behavioral intervention trial in rural Andhra Pradesh, India, conducted a 3-arm study among 600 mother-child pairs within 60 rural villages. The first arm was the control/standard of care, the second arm received an IYCN feeding intervention, and the third arm received the IYCN intervention with additional messages and skills on RF and child development. Although the intervention did not show better growth within the third arm (but did in the second arm), mental development scores in the RF group were significantly higher compared to the control and CF groups [46]. In a cohort study of 217 African-American mother-infant pairs in North Carolina, caregiver feeding style data were collected from 3 to 18 months of infant age using the Infant Feeding Style Questionnaire [47]. Parental feeding styles, including beliefs and practices, had a significant impact on both infant diet and growth, with pressuring and indulgent feeding styles associated with negative IYCF behaviors, such as greater infant energy intake, reduced odds of breastfeeding, and higher levels of age-inappropriate feeding of liquids and solids [48]. In the same study, Slining et al. [49] found that both infant overweight and high subcutaneous fat were associated with delayed infant motor development.

Future Research
In a 2013 *Lancet* article, several nutrition-specific interventions were assessed across the lifecycle [50]. This included interventions of adolescents, women of reproductive age, pregnant women, infants, and children in multiple countries. The review also assessed the design and implementation process of these nutrition interventions. The results for young children concluded that (1) community breastfeeding promotion had positive impacts on breastfeeding rates, but more data are needed on how this affects growth outcomes later in childhood; (2) previous CF interventions have been insufficient; additional trials, especially trials in food insecure populations, are needed; (3) more interventions need to be targeted toward those with moderate acute malnutrition, specifically infants younger than 6 months of age [50].

   As the global nutrition transition continues to affect changes in diet and lifestyle, research and interventions should focus on both under- and overnutrition to inform programs and policy. For infants and young children in every setting, promotion and assessment of breastfeeding and appropriate CF should be a priority. There is a clear gap of data on beverage consumption in early childhood and a need for more research, particularly as access to sugar-sweetened beverages and industry marketing continues to increase [33]. Finally, continued research on the role of caregiver feeding styles and their associations with child growth and development is needed, recognizing the importance of not just *what and when* children are fed but *how* they are fed. This research should clearly define RF components, messages, and measures, particularly within intervention studies and evaluations of programs.

Disclosure Statement

The authors have no disclosures.

References

1 Christian P, Mullany LC, Hurley KM, et al: Nutrition and maternal, neonatal, and child health. Semin Perinatol 2015;39:361–372.
2 United Nations Children's Fund (UNICEF), World Health Organization, International Bank for Reconstruction and Development/The World Bank: Levels and Trends in Child Malnutrition: Key Findings of the 2019 Edition of the Joint Child Malnutrition Estimates. Geneva, World Health Organization, 2019.
3 World Health Organization: Children: Reducing Mortality. Geneva, World Health Organization, 2018. https://www.who.int/news-room/fact-sheets/detail/children-reducing-mortality.
4 Adair LS, Popkin BM: Are child eating patterns being transformed globally? Obes Res 2005;13: 1281–1299.
5 Popkin BM: The nutrition transition and obesity in the developing world. J Nutr 2001;131:871S–873S.
6 World Health Organization: Infant and Young Child Feeding. Geneva, World Health Organization, 2018. https://www.who.int/news-room/fact-sheets/detail/infant-and-young-child-feeding.
7 United Nations Children's Fund (UNICEF): From the First Hour of Life, 2016. https://data.unicef.org/wp-content/uploads/2016/10/From-the-first-hour-of-life.pdf.
8 Victora CG, Bahl R, Barros AJ, et al: Breastfeeding in the 21st century: epidemiology, mechanisms, and lifelong effect. Lancet 2016;387:475–490.
9 Adu-Afarwuah S, Lartey A, Dewey K: Meeting nutritional needs in the first 1,000 days: A place for small-quantity lipid-based nutrient supplements. Ann N Y Acad Sci 2017;1392:18–29.
10 World Health Organization: Infant and Young Child Feeding: Model Chapter for Textbooks for Medical Students and Allied Health Professionals. Geneva, World Health Organization, 2009. https://www.who.int/nutrition/publications/infantfeeding/9789241597494/en/.
11 World Health Organization, United Nations Children's Fund: Guideline: Updates on HIV and Infant Feeding: the Duration of Breastfeeding, and Support from Health Services to Improve Feeding Practices among Mothers Living with HIV. Geneva, World Health Organization, 2016. https://apps.who.int/iris/bitstream/handle/10665/246260/9789241549707-eng.pdf?sequence = 1.
12 Chasela CS, Hudgens MG, Jamieson DJ, et al: Maternal or infant antiretroviral drugs to reduce HIV-1 transmission. N Engl J Med 2010;362: 2271–2281.
13 Tiwari S, Bharadva K, Yadav B, et al: Infant and young child feeding guidelines, 2016. Indian Pediatr 2016; 53:703–713. https://www.indianpediatrics.net/aug2016/703.pdf.
14 World Health Organization: Complementary Feeding. Geneva, World Health Organization, 2019 . https://www.who.int/nutrition/topics/complementary_feeding/en/.
15 Black MM, Aboud FE: Responsive feeding is embedded in a theoretical framework of responsive parenting. J Nutr 2011;141:490–494.
16 World Health Organization, United Nations Children's Fund, International Food Policy Research Institute: Indicators for assessing infant and young child feeding practices. Geneva, World Health Organization, 2007. https://www.who.int/maternal_child_adolescent/documents/9789241596664/en/.

17 Sriraman NK: The nuts and bolts of breastfeeding: Anatomy and physiology of lactation. Curr Probl Pediatr Adolesc Health Care 2017;47:305–310.

18 United Nations Children's Fund (UNICEF): Infant and Young Child Feeding, 2018. https://data.unicef.org/topic/nutrition/infant-and-young-child-feeding/.

19 International Institute for Population Sciences (IIPS) and ICF: National Family Health Survey (NFHS-4), 2015–16: India. Mumbai: IIPS, 2017. http://rchiips.org/nfhs/NFHS-4Reports/India.pdf.

20 International Institute for Population Sciences (IIPS) and Macro International: National Family Health Survey (NFHS-3), 2005–06: India: Volume I. Mumbai: IIPS, 2007. https://www.dhsprogram.com/pubs/pdf/FRIND3/FRIND3-Vol1%5BOct-17–2008%5D.pdf.

21 Bentley ME, Dee DL, Jensen JL: Breastfeeding among low income, African-American women: power, beliefs and decision making. J Nutr 2003; 133:305S–309S.

22 Raheel H, Tharkar S: Why mothers are not exclusively breast feeding their babies till 6 months of age? Knowledge and practices data from two large cities of the Kingdom of Saudi Arabia. Sudan J Paediatr 2018;18:28–38.

23 DiGirolamo AM, Grummer-Strawn LM, Fein SB: Do perceived attitudes of physicians and hospital staff affect breastfeeding decisions? Birth 2003; 30:94–100.

24 Radzyminski S, Callister LC: Mother's beliefs, attitudes, and decision making related to infant feeding choices. J Perinat Educ 2016;25:18–28.

25 Hunter-Adams J, Myer L, Rother HA: Perceptions related to breastfeeding and the early introduction of complementary foods amongst migrants in Cape Town, South Africa. Int Breastfeed J 2016;11:29.

26 Scott JA, Binns CW, Oddy WH, et al: Predictors of breastfeeding duration: evidence from a cohort study. Pediatrics 2006;117:e646–e55.

27 United Nations Children's Fund (UNICEF): Annual Results Report 2017 Nutrition, 2017. https://www.unicef.org/publicpartnerships/files/2017_UNICEF_ARR_Nutrition_ADVANCE_COPY.pdf.

28 Issaka AI, Agho KE, Page AN, et al: The problem of suboptimal complementary feeding practices in West Africa: what is the way forward? Maternal Child Nutr 2015;11(suppl 1):53–60.

29 Ng CS, Dibley MJ, Agho KE: Complementary feeding indicators and determinants of poor feeding practices in Indonesia: a secondary analysis of 2007 Demographic and Health Survey data. Public Health Nutr 2012;15:827–839.

30 Kabir I, Khanam M, Agho K, et al: Determinants of inappropriate complementary feeding practices in infant and young children in Bangladesh: secondary data analysis of Demographic Health Survey, 2007. Maternal Child Nutr 2012;8(Suppl 1):11–27.

31 Joshi N, Agho KE, Dibley MJ, et al: Determinants of inappropriate complementary feeding practices in young children in Nepal: Secondary data analysis of Demographic and Health survey, 2006. Maternal Child Nutr 2011;8(Suppl 1):45–59.

32 Senarath U, Godakandage SS, Jayawickrama H, et al: Determinants of inappropriate complementary feeding practices in young children in Sri Lanka: secondary data analysis of Demographic and Health Survey, 2006–2007. Matern Child Nutr 2012;8(suppl 1):60–77.

33 Dallazen C, Silva SAD, Gonçalves VSS, et al: Introduction of inappropriate complementary feeding in the first year of life and associated factors in children with low socioeconomic status. Cad Saude Publica 2018; 34:e00202816.

34 Basu S, McKee M, Galea G, Stuckler D: Relationship of soft drink consumption to global overweight, obesity, and diabetes: a cross-national analysis of 75 countries. Am J Public Health 2013; 103:2071–2077.

35 Kay MC, Welker EB, Jacquier EF, Story MT: Beverage consumption patterns among infants and young children (0–47.9 Months): data from the feeding infants and toddlers study, 2016. Nutrients 2018;10:pii:E825.

36 Kleinman RE: American academy of pediatrics recommendations for complementary feeding. Pediatrics 2000;106:1274.

37 Fledderjohann J, Doyle P, Campbell O, et al: What do Indian children drink when they do not receive water? Statistical analysis of water and alternative beverage consumption from the 2005–2006 Indian National Family Health Survey. BMC Public Health 2015;15:612.

38 Engle PL, Bentley M, Pelto G: The role of care in nutrition programmes: Current research and a research agenda. Proc Nutr Soc 2000;59:25–35.

39 Hurley KM, Cross MB, Hughes SO: A systematic review of responsive feeding and child obesity in high-income countries. J Nutr 2011;141:495–501.

40 Wasser H, Bentley M, Borja J, et al: Infants perceived as "fussy" are more likely to receive complementary foods before 4 months. Pediatrics 2011;127:229–237.

41 Thompson AL, Bentley ME: The critical period of infant feeding for the development of early disparities in obesity. Soc Sci Med 2013;97:288–296.

42 Bentley ME, Wasser HM, Creed-Kanashiro HM: Responsive feeding and child undernutrition in low- and middle-income countries. J Nutr 2011; 141:502–507.

43 Ventura AK: Associations between breastfeeding and maternal responsiveness: a systematic review of the literature. Adv Nutr 2017;8:495–510.

44 Moore AC, Akhter S, Aboud FE: Responsive complementary feeding in rural Bangladesh. Soc Sci Med 2006;62:1917–1930.

45 Abebe Z, Haki GD, Baye K: Child feeding style is associated with food intake and linear growth in rural Ethiopia. Appetite 2017;116:132–138.

46 Vazir S, Engle P, Balakrishna N, et al: Cluster-randomized trial on complementary and responsive feeding education to caregivers found improved dietary intake, growth, and development among rural Indian toddlers. Matern Child Nutr 2013;9:99–117.

47 Thompson AL, Mendez MA, Borja JB, et al: Development and validation of the infant feeding style questionnaire. Appetite 2009;53:210–221.

48 Thompson AL, Adair LS, Bentley ME: Pressuring and restrictive feeding styles influence infant feeding and size among a low-income African American sample. Obesity (Silver Spring) 2013; 21:562–571.

49 Slining M, Adair LS, Goldman BD, et al: Infant overweight is associated with delayed motor development. J Pediatr 2010;157:20–25.

50 Bhutta ZA, Das JK, Rizvi A, et al: Evidence-based interventions for improvement of maternal and child nutrition: What can be done and at what cost? Lancet 2013;382:452–477.

Michaelsen KF, Neufeld LM, Prentice AM (eds): Global Landscape of Nutrition Challenges in
Infants and Children. Nestlé Nutr Inst Workshop Ser, vol 93, pp 25–37, (DOI: 10.1159/000503354)
Nestlé Nutrition Institute, Switzerland/S. Karger AG., Basel, © 2020

Improving Children's Diet: Approach and Progress

Usha Ramakrishnan · Aimee Webb Girard

Hubert Department of Global Health, Rollins School of Public Health, Emory University, Atlanta, GA, USA

Abstract

We highlight key findings from a recent comprehensive review of social and behavior change communication (SBCC) interventions to improve complementary feeding in low-middle-income countries and discuss 4 large-scale programs as illustrative case studies. Improving dietary diversity was the most commonly targeted practice, and interpersonal communication was the most commonly used platform for the 64 interventions included in the comprehensive review. The number of behavior change techniques used by any one intervention ranged from 2 to 13 (median 6); all provided instruction on how to perform the target behavior(s), followed by the use of a "credible" source to provide the SBCC ($n = 46$), demonstration of the behavior ($n = 35$) and providing information about health consequences of the behavior ($n = 35$). The key factors that contributed to the success of the large-scale programs applying SBCC alone, or in combination with point-of-use fortification or nutrition-sensitive agriculture, included the formation of alliances with key stakeholders, availability of funds, technical support from multiple donors, well-defined theory of change, and streamlined processes for monitoring and implementation. Major limitations included a lack of detailed information on (a) intervention design, (b) behavioral theories or frameworks, (c) implementation processes including adaptations to context, and (d) cost and feasibility.

© 2020 Nestlé Nutrition Institute, Switzerland/S. Karger AG, Basel

Introduction

Despite significant strides in reducing the burden of malnutrition among young children globally, nearly 1 of 3 continues to experience linear growth retardation with short- and long-term implications for human capital and health. In parallel, the burden of overweight and obesity is a significant global public health problem, and strategies and policies that address the double or even triple burden of malnutrition that include micronutrient deficiencies among young children are needed [1]. The etiology of these conditions is complex; both immediate causes such as inadequate food, health, and care and the more distal causes that relate to the social and physical environment also need to be addressed [2]. Most notably, considerable efforts have been made by the global nutrition community to characterize and identify challenges in ensuring the adequacy of dietary intakes of young children for optimal growth and development [3].

Strategies to improve dietary intakes in young children in low-middle income countries (LMIC) have focused on both dietary quality and quantity of food consumed. While most target mothers of young children as the primary caregivers, there is an increasing recognition of the role of others in the family such as fathers and grandmothers as well as alternative settings such as day care setting (formal and informal settings) where young children are fed. A wide range of interventions aiming to improve dietary intakes of young children, have been evaluated in large-scale effectiveness trials with varying success and challenges. These interventions typically include one or more of the following targeted at infants 6–24 months of age: (a) provision of targeted food-based supplements, (b) food aid packages, (c) counseling, education, and/ or behavior change communication, (d) conditional cash transfers, (e) nutrition-sensitive interventions agriculture, (f) point-of-use fortification (micronutrient powders [MNPs]), and (g) provision of fortified products or supplements (single, multiple, lipid-based). Systematic reviews of this evidence base indicate statistically significant impacts on child growth and micronutrient status, albeit the magnitude of effects for growth is often small [4–8].

In this paper, we briefly review findings from a recent comprehensive review of interventions that used social and behavior change communication (SBCC) alone or in combination with other strategies to improve infant and young child feeding (IYCF) practices in LMIC [9]. We then identified 4 large-scale programs from sub-Saharan Africa and South/Southeast Asia as illustrative case studies for the following approaches: SBCC alone (Alive and Thrive [A&T]) and SBCC in combination with (1) point-of-use fortification (Jeevan Jyoti and Pushtikona) and (2) nutrition-sensitive agriculture (Helen Keller International [HKI] Homestead Food Production program). For each case study, we elaborate the design,

Ramakrishnan · Webb Girard

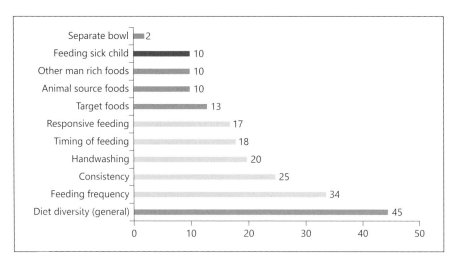

Fig. 1. Targeted complementary feeding practices (*n* = 64 interventions).

Counseling and Behavior Change Interventions

We recently completed a comprehensive review of the literature and identified 64 interventions that used SBCC strategies alone and in combination with other approaches to improve complementary feeding practices of young children [9]. The majority of interventions were conducted in South and South East Asia (*n* = 29) and sub-Saharan Africa (*n* = 22). Improving dietary diversity was the most commonly targeted practice, followed by practices related to feeding frequency, amount, responsive feeding, and handwashing (Fig. 1). Interpersonal communication, either individually or in groups, was the most commonly used platform for delivery of the SBCC strategy, followed by media (small, medium, and mass), community or social mobilization (*n* = 12), and policy advocacy/enforcement (*n* = 5). For each intervention, we systematically mapped the specific techniques used to change target behaviors as described in the available literature using the Taxonomy of Behavior Change Techniques (BCTs) developed by Abraham and Mitchie [10]. Of the 96 available techniques in the taxonomy, complementary feeding interventions collectively used a total of 28. The maximum number of techniques applied by any one intervention was 13 and the minimum 2. The median applied by any one intervention was 6. As expected, all interventions provided instruction on how to perform the behavior. Other commonly applied BCTs included use of a credible source to deliver the

SBCC intervention ($n = 46$), demonstrating the target behaviors ($n = 35$), providing information about health consequences ($n = 30$), providing social support ($n = 30$), and altering the physical or social environment (e.g., by providing food, supplements, agricultural inputs, or activities to shift social norms).

Among those BCTs used in >20 interventions, the following had effectiveness ratios >0.8: (i) providing information about the positive or negative health consequences of the behavior, (ii) demonstration of the behavior, (iii) provision of/ enabling social support, and (iv) adding objects to the environment such as food, supplements, or agricultural inputs.

From this comprehensive review of SBCC strategies to shift complementary feeding, we identified 5 large multicountry studies including A&T; Windows of Opportunity (CARE); Nutrition at the Center (CARE); Enhanced Homestead Food Production (HKI); and MICAH (World Vision). A brief description of the A&T project implementation in Ethiopia and lessons learned are summarized here.

A&T Project

From 2009 to 2014, the A&T Project, funded by the Bill and Melinda Gates Foundation and the governments of Canada and Ireland, was implemented by FHI360, in Bangladesh, Vietnam, and Ethiopia [11–13]. The A&T design and implementation framework for operating at scale includes 4 primary components related to the use of (1) mass media to support advocacy and social and behavior change; (2) interpersonal counseling and behavior change communication targeting households and influencers; (3) partnership and capacity strengthening with strategic stakeholders in implementation, monitoring, and decision-making, and (4) strategic use of monitoring, outcomes, and other data to inform advocacy and programming efforts. Formative research in each country contributed to contextually focused intervention design processes and implementation strategies. As a result, different BCTs were applied in different countries. For example, in partnership with the Ministry of Health, A&T Ethiopia focused on mobilizing families and communities to adopt 7 feeding actions (Fig. 2) and identification and social recognition of "smart and strong families" adopting these practices and "model kebeles" establishing community structures to support families in attaining this achievement. The approach to interpersonal communication and behavior change in the Ethiopia A&T project used multiple specific BCT (Table 1) as well as mass media campaigns to shift social norms on IYCF practices. Over the project period, A&T estimated that it reached approximately 2 million households with child feeding messages. A total of 4,726 households from 132 kebeles received model family certificates for achieving each of the 7 feeding actions. Evaluations noted a 5.6% decline in stunting in intervention relative to control areas as well as increased rates of exclusive

Ramakrishnan · Webb Girard

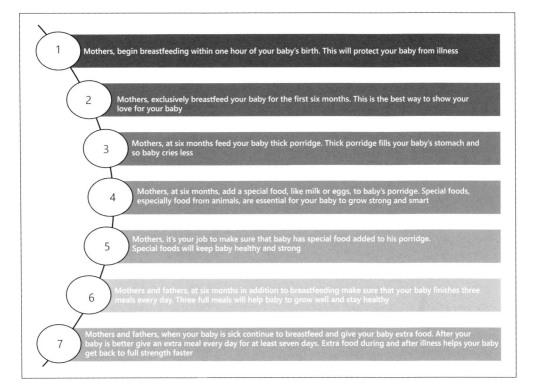

Fig. 2. Seven feeding actions – A&T, Ethiopia.

Table 1. BCT mapped to A&T

Ethiopia intervention using the taxonomy of behavior change*

1.1	Goal setting for behavior (IPC, achieving small, doable actions)
1.2	Problem solving (IPC)
2.3	Self-monitoring of behavior (strong and smart family self-assessment tool)
3.1	Social support (IPC and mass media targeting men)
4.1	Instruction on how to perform behavior (IPC and child nutrition card)
5.1	Information on positive consequences of behavior (IPC)
6.1	Demonstration of behavior (enriched porridge preparation)
9.1	Credible source (women's development army volunteers)
10.4	Social reward (smart and strong family certificate)
12.2	Restructuring social environment (mass media)
13.2	Framing/reframing

* X.Y. presented as BCT code, description (implementation of BCT).
BCT, behavior change techniques; A&T, Alive & Thrive; IPC, interpersonal communication with individualized counseling.

breastfeeding to 6 months, improved diet diversity, and increases in the proportion consuming a minimally acceptable diet.

The often overlooked components of community and policy advocacy were pivotal to the success of the A&T project at scale in all implementing countries. This multidimensional approach engaged influential and respected civil society organizations to support a more enabling policy environment for IYCF, notably women's associations in Ethiopia are directly engaged with government stakeholders, including the ministerial Office of Women, Youth and Child Affairs. In Vietnam, in addition to women's associations, A&T engaged medical profession associations to advocate for optimal IYCF, especially related to breastfeeding. A second contributor to success was the heavy investment in a robust data-driven approach, including collection, use, and application to ensure data-driven intervention design and results-based project monitoring, management, learning, and adaptation.

Home-Based Fortification Strategies
MNPs are single-serve sachets containing a mix of powdered vitamins and minerals that can be easily sprinkled once daily onto many different types of foods without changing the color, taste, or texture of the food. They were originally developed for pediatric use and have since been evaluated extensively in efficacy trials that have shown significant reductions in the burden of anemia and iron deficiency in many low-middle income settings around the world [14]. This has led to the adoption of this approach as part of large-scale programs in many countries with varying degrees of success and challenges [15]. Two case studies examining the effectiveness of MNPs as a strategy to reduce anemia and improve IYCF practices in South Asia are described here.

Jeevan-Jyothi
This project was implemented as part of a larger project Integrated Family Health Initiative that was carried out by CARE India and several other partners in 8 districts in Bihar, India. The home fortification project was a collaboration between Emory University and CARE, India, and was conducted in the district of West Champaran in Bihar, India, from 2010 to 2016. The primary goal was to evaluate the feasibility and benefits of combining home fortification using MNPs with improved counseling on IYCF practices as an approach to improve dietary intakes and child growth and reduce anemia in young children (6–24 months of age), using existing government health and Integrated Child Development Scheme functionaries [16]. Briefly, several rounds of formative research were first conducted to help contextualize the intervention. These included activities that evaluated the acceptability of the product by various stakeholders (frontline community workers, village leaders, caregivers), suitability of the packaging and

delivery platforms for the MMPs, and appropriate messages for promoting optimal IYCF practices as well as use of the MMPs [17]. The MNP powder was branded as "Jeevan Jyothi", which means "Light of my Life" and contained several key micronutrients including iron. The formative phase was followed by the pilot study in which 70 communities from 4 blocks (administrative unit within districts in India) in West Champaran District were randomized to receive the MMP intervention or not for 1 year. All communities received IYCF counseling from the frontline workers (FLWs) who also distributed the MMPs (frequency) in half the communities. As part of the evaluation, cross-sectional surveys were conducted at baseline, midline, and endline along with ongoing process monitoring that included various checklists and use of qualitative methods such as focus groups and key informant interviews. At the beginning of the program, 72 and 53% of households reported receiving and consuming MNPs, respectively, but these numbers declined to 40 and 43% at midline, respectively. Qualitative data indicated high community acceptance of MNPs and a good understanding of the program by FLWs but the key barriers to use by households were a lack of MNPs, due in part to infrequent FLW distribution, as well as perceived side effects that were addressed by revised recommendations for use. The use of real-time program data allowed for the timely identification of key program issues and appropriate decision-making to improve program implementation [16]. Furthermore, the quasi-experimental design of this project was useful to evaluate outcomes including measures of motor and mental development that improved significantly in the MNP group compared to the control [16, 18].

Pushtikona

This project is a large-scale, community-based MNP project that is being carried out in Bangladesh as a private-public partnership that was formed in 2010. This project uses a market-based approach and sought to create sustainable market mechanism and ensure access for poor and promote home fortification with MNPs in the broader context of optimum complementary feeding [19]. It comprised 3 components: building an enabling policy environment to create a supportive stakeholder and enabling policy environment for home fortification and MNP use at scale; accelerating growth in mass effective coverage through expanded delivery channels; and scaling up home fortification and demand for MNPs as a part of optimal IYCF practices. Pushtikona, a multi-MNP that contains 15 essential minerals and vitamins, was developed by the Sprinkles Global Health Initiative to prevent and treat micronutrient deficiencies in young children and other vulnerable groups and manufactured by Renata Ltd. in Bangladesh. The distribution of the sprinkles is being implemented by BRAC, the largest NGO in world that originated in Bangladesh, in partnership with the Government of Bangladesh, to ensure equal access for the most marginalized and vulnerable communities with technical support from the International Center for Diarrhoeal Disease Research, Bangladesh, A&T Project, and the Global Alliance for Improved Nutrition (GAIN). In collaboration with Renata Ltd. and GAIN who provided technical support and capital for production and marketing, BRAC is implementing the MNP program in 64 districts in Bangladesh through their network of 80,000 healthcare workers known as *Shasthya Shebika (SS)*, who sell a basket of essential social products door to door. To support their sprinkles program, BRAC has also undertaken to develop awareness of the need for fortified and nutrient-rich food and promote Pushtikona as a product. This is a multiactor approach, trying to reach mothers, caregivers, health professionals, community health workers, and other influencers. The overall program goal was to significantly improve nutritional status and reduce iron deficiency anemia by 10% among infants and children and to protect and promote optimal IYCF practices (including breastfeeding). During the first phase (2009–2014), the program reached about 100,000,000 of 160,000,000 population that included 200,000 infants and young children through retail sales alone in initial 5 years (2009–2014). In 2013, Renata manufactured 34 million sachets and the BRAC frontline workers delivered 14.5 million sachets. However, several challenges were identified (see below) in the second phase (2014–2018) of this program [15] and GAIN has helped catalyze the scale up and utilization of MNPs by children from 6 to 59 months of age to cover approximately 4 million children over a period of 5 years.

- Stock outs of MNPs from SSs
- Limited home visits by SSs in households with children under 5 years
- Lack of confidence in SSs during the promotion of MNPs at the community level
- Poor household level compliance: intrahousehold disparities and gender issues play a dominant role in compliance and buying behavior
- Perceived lack of need for MNPs among caregivers: quality, quantity, and frequency of complementary foods given to infants often inadequate to meet their increasing iron required

Leyvraz et al. [15] recently evaluated the success of home fortification programs in LMIC using the Fortification Assessment Coverage Tool that reports coverage at 3 levels, namely, (a) message coverage: awareness of the product; (b) contact coverage: use of the product ≥1 time; and (c) effective coverage: regular use aligned with program-specific goal [20]. They found considerable variation, and typically, effective coverage was very low and/or declined over time in many of these programs. In Bangladesh, message coverage ranged from 45 to 64% across the different survey rounds, whereas contact coverage reduced by nearly half (24–37%) and effective coverage was <5% in all rounds. In contrast, message and contact coverage rates were much higher (>80%) in Ghana and India where

Table 2. Range of design and implementation strategies in nutrition-sensitive agriculture

Macro-level strategies	Local strategies
Investment in rural development and agricultural sciences	Home gardens/animal husbandry programs
Policies to support nutrition-sensitive agriculture	Urban/community agriculture projects
Monitoring the food environment	Home-based food-processing techniques
Rethinking globalization, free trade, and food as profit	Community kitchens
Public-private partnerships and corporate responsibility	Irrigation projects
Land redistribution	
Markets' and value chains' infrastructure	

they were also able to attain over 50% of effective coverage. The programs in Cote D'Ivoire and Vietnam had much lower rates and all categories of coverage declined dramatically over time in Ghana. Furthermore, when they examined the extent to which the program was taken up by those presumed to be at higher risk of inadequate dietary intake that is, living in poverty and having children with suboptimal IYCF, greater disparities were observed. For example, in Bangladesh, all measures of coverage were significantly lower among those with suboptimal IYCF with no differences by poverty. Examination of barriers revealed both supply- and demand-related factors. Specifically interruptions in the availability of the product, perceived side effects, and the lack or poorly designed SBCC strategies to create demand were common. These findings clearly indicate the need for sustained support of these programs both for implementation, especially the SBCC strategies and ongoing monitoring and evaluation.

Food-Based Strategies
The importance of the social and physical environment in enabling caregivers to optimally feed young children has long been recognized as an integral component of the conceptual framework for child nutrition [2]. Increasingly, complementary feeding interventions are addressing these underlying social and physical determinants in their design and implementation. These "nutrition-sensitive" interventions aim to improve access to nutritious food while addressing the other underlying determinants of poor nutrition such as water and sanitation and women's empowerment [21]. For the purposes of this review, we focus on *nutrition-sensitive agriculture strategies*. These range in focus from the macro-level market-based strategies to micro-level, household-level strategies (Table 2).

Evidence to date suggests that nutrition-sensitive agriculture can promote more optimal complementary feeding practices, with the majority of the evidence base deriving from effectiveness studies of household-level production interventions on family and child diets [21–23]. Effectiveness strengthens in the presence of nutrition-focused SBCC and strategies to empower women [23–25]. Beyond diets, nutrition-sensitive agriculture can have impacts on health and nutritional status if they incorporate health-seeking and promote appropriate water, sanitation, and hygiene practices. For vulnerable families and in contexts where animal source foods are limited, micronutrient-rich supplemental foods or supplements, for example, MNPs, lipid-based nutritional supplements, or the provision of animal source foods such as milk or eggs, may be necessary to optimize benefits.

One programmatic case study with perhaps the longest history of success at scale is HKI's HFP program [26]. Now implemented in several countries including Nepal, Bangladesh, and Burkina Faso, the HFP program works with community partners to establish model farms and support women in homestead food production, including production of home- and market-desired fruits and vegetables, and micro-livestock such as poultry and small ruminants. Trained volunteers provide SBCC focused on nutrition and health and, in some contexts such as Burkina Faso, facilitate women's empowerment activities that promote increased access to and control over economic assets and inputs into decision-making for women. The HFP program also recognizes the limitations of local food production in specific contexts. In Nepal, for example, the HFP program implemented MNPs for vulnerable households delivered through the agricultural platform [27, 28]. Collectively, evaluations have noted enhanced status of women, increased dietary diversity, and consumption of target foods and improved micronutrient status of children [22, 26]. In Burkina Faso, enhanced HFP programs, with greater targeting of the 1,000-day window, intensive nutrition-focused SBCC and activities that promote women's empowerment, noted significantly reduced anemia and wasting in children and enhanced weight gain in women [29–31].

Despite progress made in their implementation and evaluation [23], nutrition-sensitive agriculture approaches, due to their complex and integrated nature, are fraught with challenges. Most notably, these strategies require the commitment and engagement of multiple different sectors spanning, for example, agriculture, health, rural development, or urban planning as well as public-private partnerships. Under increasing climate variability, these approaches will inevitably become more challenging and require increased resources and extension with regard to adapted seeds, irrigation systems, pest management, and safety nets. Monitoring and evaluating the costs, impact, and sustainability of these approaches on the diets, nutrition, and health of young children are complex due to the varied inputs and myriad pathways to impact. Given the multi-component nature of these interventions and their costs, the need to estimate the relative costs and contributions of the different components of integrated nutrition-sensitive interventions further complicate their evaluation. Lastly, the bulk of the evidence based on nutrition-sensitive agriculture resides with homestead food production. However, other systems' focused strategies may be as critical as homestead food production to facilitate families' access to nutritious, safe, and secure food, especially in urban and rapidly urbanizing contexts where dependence on markets for food dominates. Recent efforts have been made to expand beyond household food production and to understand and describe the food environment, markets and value chains, and food systems and their relationship to dietary intakes and nutritional status. These include efforts to develop and validate reliable assessment metrics for food environments, value chains, and food security [23]. However, improved tools are still needed that evaluate the ability of local diets to meet dietary requirements of young children.

Summary

Considerable progress has been made in identifying effective strategies that can be implemented to improve child dietary intakes in varied settings. More recently, several large at-scale programs have aimed to improve child dietary intakes in LMIC using a variety of strategies that combine one or more of the following, namely, (a) BCTs, (b) provision of enabling social support, and/or (c) adding objects to the environment such as food, supplements, or agricultural inputs. However, the lack of reporting detail has implications for the adoption, replication, and scale up of effective strategies. Similarly, there is limited information on costs and scalability. Finally, the rapid transition to obesogenic environments and increasing disparities poses additional challenges that need to be addressed while still addressing the issues of inadequate dietary intakes and/or poor dietary quality that is seen at both ends of the spectrum, that is, under- and overnutrition. For all of the approaches illustrated in these case studies, political instability, lack of accountability and transparency, and conflict in combination with the nutrition and health implications of climate change exacerbate the challenges inherent in large-scale nutrition programs, especially multisectoral ones. The role of sustained advocacy to ensure the development, adoption, and enforcement of policies that support improved child nutrition cannot be understated.

Disclosure Statement

This work was supported by a grant from the Bill and Melinda Gates Foundation and the Tata-Cornell Institute (TCI)TARINA program.

References

1 Black RE, Victora CG, Walker SP, et al: Maternal and child undernutrition and overweight in low-income and middle-income countries. Lancet 2013;382:427–451.

2 Strategy for Improved Nutrition for Children and Women in Developing Countries. New York, UNICEF, 1990.

3 White JM, Begin F, Kumapley R, et al: Complementary feeding practices: Current global and regional estimates. Matern Child Nutr 2017; 13(suppl 2).

4 Dewey KG, Adu-Afarwuah S: Systematic review of the efficacy and effectiveness of complementary feeding interventions in developing countries. Matern Child Nutr 2008; 4(suppl 1):24–85.

5 Graziose MM, Downs SM, O'Brien Q, et al: Systematic review of the design, implementation and effectiveness of mass media and nutrition education interventions for infant and young child feeding. Public Health Nutr 2018;21:273–287.

6 Lamstein S, Stillman T, Koniz-Booher P, et al: Evidence of Effective Approaches to Social and Behavior Change Communication for Preventing and Reducing Stunting and Anemia: Report from a Systematic Literature Review. Arlington, USAID/ Strengthening Partnerships, Results and Innovations in Nutrition Globally (SPRING) Project, 2014.

7 Lassi ZS, Das JK, Zahid G, et al: Impact of education and provision of complementary feeding on growth and morbidity in children less than 2 years of age in developing countries: a systematic review. BMC Public Health 2013;13(suppl 3):S13.

8 Heidkamp RA: Evidence for the effects of complementary feeding interventions on the growth of infants and young children in low- and middle-income countries. Nestle Nutr Inst Workshop Ser 2017;87:89–102.

9 Webb Girard A, Waugh E, Sawyer S, et al: A scoping review of social-behaviour change techniques applied in complementary feeding interventions. Matern Child Nutr 2019:e12882.

10 Abraham C, Michie S: A taxonomy of behavior change techniques used in interventions. Health Psychol 2008;27:379–387.

11 Kim SS, Ali D, Kennedy A, et al: Assessing implementation fidelity of a community-based infant and young child feeding intervention in Ethiopia identifies delivery challenges that limit reach to communities: a mixed-method process evaluation study. BMC Public Health 2015;15:316.

12 Menon P, Nguyen PH, Saha KK, et al: Combining intensive counseling by frontline workers with a nationwide mass media campaign has large differential impacts on complementary feeding practices but not on child growth: results of a cluster-randomized program evaluation in Bangladesh. J Nutr 2016;146:2075–2084.

13 Rawat R, Nguyen PH, Tran LM, et al: Social franchising and a nationwide mass media campaign increased the prevalence of adequate complementary feeding in Vietnam: a cluster-randomized program. J Nutr 2017;147:670–679.

14 De-Regil LM, Jefferds ME, Pena-Rosas JP: Point-of-use fortification of foods with micronutrient powders containing iron in children of preschool and school-age. Cochrane Database Syst Rev 2017;11:CD009666.

15 Leyvraz M, Aaron GJ, Poonawala A, et al: Coverage of nutrition interventions intended for infants and young children varies greatly across programs: Results from coverage surveys in 5 countries. J Nutr 2017;147:995S–1003S.

16 Mehta R, Martorell R, Chaudhuri I, et al: Use of monitoring data to improve implementation of a home fortification program in Bihar, India. Matern Child Nutr 2019;15:e12753.

17 Young MF, Kekre P, Verma P, et al: Community acceptability and utilization of micronutrient powders in Bihar, India. Faseb J 2013;27. https://www.fasebj.org/doi/abs/10.1096/fasebj.27.1_supplement.lb271.

18 Larson LM, Young MF, Bauer PJ, et al: Effectiveness of a home fortification programme with multiple micronutrients on infant and young child development: a cluster-randomised trial in rural Bihar, India. Br J Nutr 2018;120: 176–187.

19 Afsana K, Haque MR, Sobhan S, et al: BRAC's experience in scaling-up MNP in Bangladesh. Asia Pac J Clin Nutr 2014;23:377–384.

20 Friesen VM, Aaron GJ, Myatt M, et al: Assessing coverage of population-based and targeted fortification programs with the use of the fortification assessment coverage toolkit (FACT): background, toolkit development, and supplement overview. J Nutr 2017;147:981S–983S.

21 Ruel MT, Alderman H; Maternal and Child Nutrition Study Group: Nutrition-sensitive interventions and programmes: How can they help to accelerate progress in improving maternal and child nutrition? Lancet 2013;382:536–551.

22 Girard AW, Self JL, McAuliffe C, et al: The effects of household food production strategies on the health and nutrition outcomes of women and young children: a systematic review. Paediatr Perinat Epidemiol 2012;26(suppl 1):205–222.

23 Ruel MT: New Evidence on Nutrition-sensitive Agricultural Programs, Washington, International Food Policy Research Institute (IFPRI), 2019.

24 Berti PR, Krasevec J, FitzGerald S: A review of the effectiveness of agriculture interventions in improving nutrition outcomes. Public Health Nutr 2004;7:599–609.

25 Gillespie SJ, Hodge S, Yosef S, Pandya-Lorch R: Nourishing Millions: Stories of Change in Nutrition. Washington, DC: International Food Policy Research Institute (IFPRI), 2016. http://dx.doi.org/10.2499/9780896295889.

26 Haselow NJ, Stormer A, Pries A: Evidence-based evolution of an integrated nutrition-focused agriculture approach to address the underlying determinants of stunting. Matern Child Nutr 2016; 12(suppl 1):155–168.

27 Osei AK, Pandey P, Spiro D, et al: Adding multiple micronutrient powders to a homestead food production programme yields marginally significant benefit on anaemia reduction among young children in Nepal. Matern Child Nutr 2015; 11(suppl 4):188–202.

28 Osei A, Pandey P, Nielsen J, et al: Combining home garden, poultry, and nutrition education program targeted to families with young children improved anemia among children and anemia and underweight among nonpregnant women in Nepal. Food Nutr Bull 2017;38:49–64.

29 Olney DK, Talukder A, Iannotti LL, et al: Assessing impact and impact pathways of a homestead food production program on household and child nutrition in Cambodia. Food Nutr Bull 2009;30: 355–369.

30 Olney DK, Pedehombga A, Ruel MT, et al: A 2-year integrated agriculture and nutrition and health behavior change communication program targeted to women in Burkina Faso reduces anemia, wasting, and diarrhea in children 3–12.9 months of age at baseline: a cluster-randomized controlled trial. J Nutr 2015;145:1317–1324.

31 Olney DK, Bliznashka L, Pedehombga A, et al: A 2-year integrated agriculture and nutrition program targeted to mothers of young children in Burkina Faso reduces underweight among mothers and increases their empowerment: a cluster-randomized controlled trial. J Nutr 2016;146: 1109–1117.

Michaelsen KF, Neufeld LM, Prentice AM (eds): Global Landscape of Nutrition Challenges in Infants and Children. Nestlé Nutr Inst Workshop Ser, vol 93, pp 39–49, (DOI: 10.1159/000503355)
Nestlé Nutrition Institute, Switzerland/S. Karger AG., Basel, © 2020

The Importance of Food Composition Data for Estimating Micronutrient Intake: What Do We Know Now and into the Future?

Fernanda Grande[a] · Anna Vincent[b]

[a]Food and Agriculture Organization of the United Nations (FAO), São Paulo, Brazil; [b]Food and Agriculture Organization of the United Nations (FAO), Kensington Gardens, SA, Australia

Abstract

Food composition tables and databases (FCT/FCDB) centralize data on the energy and nutrient content of foods of a certain country or region. They are essential for many activities related to nutrition. The main factors that can affect the quality of FCT/FCDB are the sources of the data, coverage of foods and components, food description, and component identification. Around 100 countries have published at least one FCT/FCDB, although many of them are outdated and vary considerably in terms of data quality, documentation, and accessibility. A great number of those FCT/FCDB contain very few up-to-date analytical data obtained for food composition purposes, resulting in many data being estimated or copied from publicly available FCT/FCDB from other countries. In addition, many other natural factors that can affect the composition of foods are often not reflected in FCT/FCDB, including biodiversity, maturation degree, soil, and harvest season. Therefore, the use of low-quality FCT/FCDB to convert food consumption data into energy and nutrient intakes may introduce errors resulting in under- or overestimated intake for a certain component. These wrong conclusions may lead to inappropriate or inefficient nutrition and health-related policies, especially to improve micronutrient status in populations and individuals.

© 2020 Nestlé Nutrition Institute, Switzerland/S. Karger AG, Basel

Introduction

Reducing all forms of malnutrition represents a great challenge in many countries, and high-quality data on population nutrient intakes are required to solve this problem. In this context, food composition tables and databases (FCT/FCDB) are an essential tool for dietary assessment as they provide the information required to convert food consumption data into energy and nutrient intakes [1–3].

FCT/FCDB centralize data on the nutrient content of foods of a certain country or region. In addition to their use in dietary assessment, FCT/FCDB are the basis for many activities involving nutrition and health, food security, and agriculture [1, 3–5].

Energy and nutrient intakes are calculated by matching foods consumed with data from FCT/FCDB. Understanding the potential sources of error in FCT/FCDB is important as these errors affect the calculation of intakes [1, 6]; the more accurately FCT/FCDB reflect the foods actually consumed, the better quality the intake estimates will be. This paper discusses the quality and availability of global FCT/FCDB, important considerations for their use and current challenges and opportunities in food composition.

FCT/FCDB: Sources of Data

Data in FCT/FCDB come from these main sources, in general order of quality and preference [7]:
- Analytical data, either from food composition-specific sampling programs or scientific journals, research data, or laboratory reports (e.g., from food industry)
- Imputed values
- Recipe calculations
- Data borrowed from other FCT/FCDB
- Presumed values

Food composition-specific sampling programs analyze representative samples across a country or region so that they accurately reflect the food supply. These data are considered the highest quality data [7], although it is important that they are up-to-date. Published data from scientific journals, research data, and laboratory reports are usually of sound analytical quality but may represent only a small subset of available foods, for example, a particular variety of plant, or foods from a small region. In particular, data for processed foods (often from industry) are important in keeping FCT/FCDB current, as reformulation is frequent and can significantly change composition.

Imputed values are data taken from similar foods (e.g., values for spinach used for other dark green leafy vegetables). Use of these values relies on good food composition knowledge and an understanding of the food to ensure values appropriate to impute.

Recipe calculations are generally used to estimate the composition of cooked foods, either single foods or mixed dishes, where analytical data exist only for the raw form. Recipes use nutrient retention factors to estimate the loss of nutrients and yield factors to estimate the change in water (and sometimes also fat) during cooking [8].

Borrowed data are used where local data are not available. Data need to be scrutinized to ensure that they match foods consumed locally, for example, for fortification, trimming practices for meat, local consumption patterns such as the addition of salt to cooked foods, color of fruit and vegetables, and so on. Given the wide range of factors that can affect food composition, there will always be uncertainty around the applicability of borrowed data and its use should be limited [8].

Many components can be presumed zero based on existing knowledge or food composition research; for example, dietary fiber in meat, poultry, milk, fish, and eggs and retinol and cholesterol in unfortified plant products [9].

Most FCT/FCDB contain values from all these sources since it represents the most cost-effective method of preparing FCT/FCDB. The best approach to initiate a food composition program is to directly analyze staple foods and take data for less important foods from other sources when necessary. A reliable FCT/FCDB should also have a limited number of imputed and calculated values [7].

Limitations and Quality Considerations for Using FCT/FCDB

The composition of a food may change due to a number of reasons, such as intrinsic (e.g., variety or cultivar) and extrinsic factors (e.g., farming conditions). However, differences in nutrient contents between FCT/FCDB may also be due to the quality of the data, analytical methods used, or ways of expressing the nutrient. Identifying these factors, which are summarized in Table 1, is of great importance to avoid incorrect uses and comparisons.

Variability in the Composition of Foods
Since foods are biological materials, natural variation in their nutrient content is expected [7]. Many factors that may affect the nutrient content, including biodiversity, maturation degree, and harvest season, are often not reflected in FCT/FCDB.

The variation in the nutrient content between distinct varieties or cultivars of the same species can represent the difference between nutrient deficiency and

Table 1. Limitations and considerations for using Food Composition Tables and Databases [7]

Variability in the composition of foods
    Inherent (variety/cultivar/breed, maturity/age, color)
    Environmental (soil, water, weather, sunlight, fertilizer, feed)
    Transport and storage (time, temperature, light)
    Removal/addition of components (e.g., fat removal or nutrient fortification)
    Processing/preparation
    Product or recipe formulation

Limited coverage of food items and components
    Food items or components of interest are not included, especially processed foods
    Missing values (results in underestimates of nutrient intakes)

Inappropriate database or food composition values
    Lack of analytical data obtained for food composition purposes
    Out-of-date data

Errors arising in database use
    Incorrect food matching
    Mistakes in nutrient definitions, units, and conversions
    Wrong procedures for recipe calculations

Incompatibility of databases
    Different analytical methods, definitions, and modes of expression ("problematic"
    components include energy, protein, fat, carbohydrate, dietary fiber, vitamins A,
    D, E, K, C, folate, and niacin)

---

nutrient adequacy in populations and individuals. For instance, vitamin A content in sweet potato may vary from trace amounts to 3,637 µg retinol equivalents (RE) per 100 g of edible portion [10], which is 6 times the recommended daily intake for this nutrient [11]. Flesh color indicates the vitamin A content as yellow- and orange-fleshed sweet potatoes contain higher amounts of vitamin A. Hence, these foods should be reported individually in FCT/FCDB with their unique nutrient profile instead of a singular food entry with an average value [12].

The nutrient content of plant foods may also change during ripening. An increase in the vitamin A content has been found in several fruits and vegetables such as mango, papaya, cabbage, and lettuce due to enhanced carotenogenesis [13]. In contrast, vitamin C content generally decreases in fruits as a consequence of the metabolic stress during ripening, which requires antioxidant action to prevent cell damage [14].

In addition, climate change may also affect food composition. Meta-analyses have considered the impacts of increased CO_2, water stress, and higher temperatures on nutrient composition in plant foods [15, 16]. Particular attention has been given to the effect of increased CO_2 on staple crops such as wheat; a 2017 meta-analysis reports that for wheat, increasing CO_2 in the atmosphere decreases the concentration of protein and some minerals (including, importantly, iron and zinc) [16]. For food growers, adapting to climate change may require new plant varieties; as discussed above, there can be large differences in the composition between different varieties. The impact of climate change on nutrient content of foods is just one of the reasons FCT/FCDB need to be updated regularly so that data accurately reflect the current food supply.

Quality of FCT/FCDB

The main factors that affect the quality of FCT/FCDB are the sources of food composition data (discussed at FCT/FCDB: Sources of Data), coverage of foods and components, and details included in the food description and component identification (including denominators, units, and definitions).

A good quality FCT/FCDB should include the foods consumed by the person or population of interest [6, 17]. Therefore, FCT/FCDB need to be regularly updated to reflect changes in the food supply and nutrition science [2]. Many FCT/FCDB do not include fortified foods (voluntary or mandatory), commercially processed foods, mixed dishes, or an accurate representation of the biodiverse foods consumed by the population of interest. For instance, nearly 60 countries have legislation mandating fortification of corn and/or wheat flours with folic acid [18]. However, only 10 of those countries have published FCT/FCDB, which include data on folate, and just 6 also include fortified foods. As a result, some dietary assessments post fortification have failed to include fortified foods in their calculated micronutrient intakes [1], meaning that the true intake was possibly underestimated.

FCT/FCDB require detailed food names/descriptions to accurately match food composition data to foods consumed. Nutrient contents can differ greatly, for example, between raw and cooked versions of the same food and between different parts of an edible plant or animal. In the 2012 West African FCT, rice (white, polished, raw) has an energy value of 1,500 kJ per 100 g of edible portion; rice (white, polished, boiled [without salt]) has only 580 kJ per 100 g of edible portion [19]. For cassava, the raw leaves contain 286 µg of vitamin A, retinol activity equivalent (RAE) per 100 g of edible portion, whereas the raw tuber contains 1 µg of vitamin A, RAE per 100 g of edible portion. Therefore, food names should include important details such as cooking and preservation method, color and form, variety/cultivar/breed, maturity, origin, part of the animal or plant, edible/inedible portion, and fortification or enrichment since these may affect the nutrient content of foods [8].

FCT/FCDB should include complete data for nutrients of interest; missing nutrient data require the user to estimate or borrow data, otherwise nutrient intakes will be underestimated.

Clear and complete descriptions of the components presented are important to the quality of FCT/FCDB and to ensure "like for like" comparisons with recommended dietary intakes or between nutrient intake studies and different FCT/FCDBs. Details should include:

– Analytical methods used; since for some components (e.g., dietary fiber, folate, vitamin C and phytate) different analytical methods give different values for the same foods.
– How the data are expressed, for example, amino acids can be expressed per 100 g edible portion of food, or per g of nitrogen; fatty acids can be expressed per 100 g edible portion of food or as a fraction of total fatty acids.
– Which specific chemical entities the component name covers, for example, vitamin E can be defined as alpha-tocopherol only or calculated from multiple tocopherols and tocotrienols.
– Whether the component is derived by calculation and if so, how it is calculated including unit and conversion factors used, if applicable. For example, total vitamin A may be calculated either as RE or as RAE, and in plant foods, they result in different values for the same carotenoid content. Thus, using RE or RAE in estimating nutrient intake would generate 2 significantly different figures [20]. Similar problems may occur for other components, for example, niacin and folate.

Given the number of factors that can affect the composition of foods and the diversity of the food supply and individual consumption patterns, even the highest quality FCT/FCDB will not represent all foods available in a certain region. Thus, it is important that all users are aware of limitations and considerations for using FCT/FCDB, since they can affect intake estimates.

Global Availability of FCT/FCDB

According to global inventories [21], >100 countries have published at least one FCT/FCDB already. However, about 90 countries still have no published national FCT/FCDB, mostly middle- and low-income countries (Fig. 1). Even where countries have published FCT/FCDB, many are composed of incomplete and unreliable data [22]. These countries borrow data from publicly available FCT/FCDB, while this information should be developed at country level, regardless of their land extension. Even in small countries, the composition of foods may differ from other countries due to plant and animal varieties consumed, environmental conditions, soil composition, agricultural practices, fortification programs, product formulation, and dietary habits [2, 23]. Adapting FCT/FCDB from another country can be challenging and time-consuming due

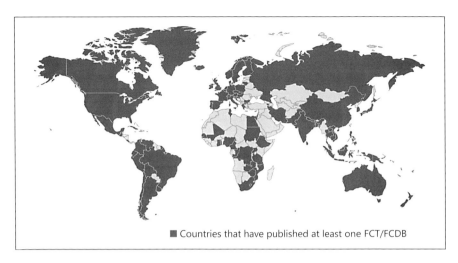

Fig. 1. Countries with published national Food Composition Table or Database (FCT/FCDB) as on December 2018 [21].

to these differences in the food items. For instance, a comparison of the micro-nutrient content in Brazilian foods with the FCDB from the United States Department of Agriculture showed large differences in the content of some minerals and vitamin A [20, 24]. Thus, using this FCDB to estimate nutrient intake in Brazil may lead to wrong conclusions when evaluating micronutrient adequacy.

Figure 2 shows FCT/FCDB published before December 2018, according to the different regions and to the number of years since last update. Out of the 107 FCT/FCDB available, 52 (49%) were published or had their last update >10 years ago. Most outdated FCT/FCDB are in Africa, followed by Latin America and Europe. The lack of reliable national FCT/FCDB is among the major limitations for dietary assessment in Africa [25], since half of the countries in this continent have never published FCT/FCDB, while the others have only outdated versions. The low frequency of updates of those FCT/FCDB is due to the scarcity of resources required to carry out this complex task [22].

Published FCT/FCDB vary considerably in terms of data quality, documentation, food and nutrient coverage, analytical methods used, and accessibility [2]. Unfortunately, many FCT/FCDB include data only for a limited number of components and for a small number of raw foods, while mixed dishes and foods that are cooked, processed, or fortified are often lacking [22]. Those FCT/FCDB also contain very few up-to-date analytical data obtained for food composition purposes, resulting in many data being estimated or copied from other publicly available FCT/FCDB [3]. For example, some FCT/FCDB from countries in sub-Saharan Africa borrow up to 88% of all data for animal-source foods, mainly from high-income countries [26].

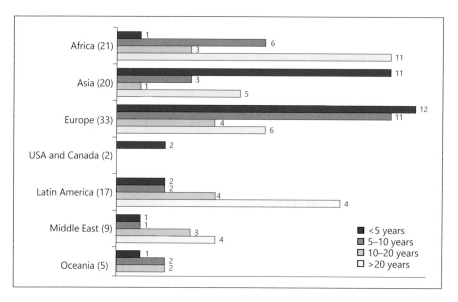

Fig. 2. Food composition tables and databases (FCT/FCDB) listed in global inventories [21] in December 2018 by region and according to the number of years since last update. Values in parentheses correspond to the total number of FCT/FCDB available in the region.

Even though many FCT/FCDB still need to be published or updated, about 30 countries have published or updated their FCT/FCDB in the past 5 years. These activities were developed in all regions, but the majority belong to countries in Europe and Asia (Fig. 2). A successful example is the latest version of the Indian FCT, launched in 2017. This version includes solely new analytical data for over 500 raw foods sampled by a statistically valid sampling method and collected from the different regions of the country. The update added 136 new components compared to the previous edition from 1989, resulting in about 200 components presented for all new foods [27].

The increasing interest in food composition in the recent years is probably due also to the efforts of international initiatives in advocating for the need of reliable FCT/FCDB [3].

Global Initiatives, Challenges, and Opportunities

The International Network of Food Data Systems (INFOODS) was established in 1984 to coordinate food composition activities aiming to improve data quality and availability globally. This international network is structured into regional data centers that have national branches. These are headed by a global coordinator (since 1999 at FAO) and regional coordinators [4].

INFOODS' activities include capacity development and publication of both guidelines and regional and international FCT/FCDB that are available on their website free-of-charge [4]. The e-Learning Course on Food Composition Data represents an important tool to raise awareness of the importance of food composition among professionals working with these data. This online training course can be accessed from the FAO website providing a deeper knowledge on food composition data principles and processes for both students and professionals [28].

Many FCT/FCDB were developed under the regional or national INFOODS data centers, especially in high-income countries. An example is the former European Network of Food Data Systems, which has become the European Food Information Resource (EuroFIR). The main objective of EuroFIR is to create and disseminate a standardized and reliable source of food composition data for different uses across Europe. To assist food composition data compilers, EuroFIR has also produced a range of tools and standards to support the exchange and comparison of data in European countries [5].

Despite these international initiatives, publishing or updating FCT/FCDB remains a challenge for many countries. A major obstacle is the lack of an institutional "home" for ongoing FCT/FCDB activities, once an initial table has been published. Continuing national food composition programs are fundamental for maintaining the currency of FCT/FCDB and ensuring they accurately represent the foods currently being consumed by the population. In countries where there is no food composition program, even if new composition data of local foods is generated and published for research purposes, they are not captured and included into the national FCT/FCDB [29].

Developing high-quality FCT/FCDB is costly and time-consuming and also requires analytical laboratories, facilities, and trained professionals. Thus, to provide country-specific data in FCT/FCDB, there is a need to combine efforts from different sectors, such as government, universities, researchers, and the private sector to gather local food composition data [3]. Partnerships between government and research institutes can result in significant developments in national FCT/FCDB [23]. These investments also need to be cost-effective, scientifically robust, and effectively result in stakeholder awareness and engagement [5].

Concluding Remarks

Despite food composition receiving more attention in recent years, many countries still need to generate and disseminate up-to-date and high-quality FCT/FCDB due to the significance of this information. Poor food composition data may lead to wrong conclusions resulting in the development of misleading policies and programs in nutrition to improve the nutritional status, especially for micronutrients, of individuals and populations.

Disclosure Statement

The authors have no conflicts of interest to declare.

References

1 Gibson RS, Charrondiere UR, Bell W: Measurement errors in dietary assessment using self-reported 24-hour recalls in low-income countries and strategies for their prevention. Adv Nutr 2017;8:980–991.
2 Ene-Obong H, Schönfeldt HC, Campaore E, et al: Importance and use of reliable food composition data generation by nutrition/dietetic professionals towards solving Africa's nutrition problem: constraints and the role of FAO/INFOODS/AFROFOODS and other stakeholders in future initiatives. Proc Nutr Soc 2019; 78:496–505.
3 Micha R, Coates J, Leclercq C, et al: Global dietary surveillance: data gaps and challenges. Food Nutr Bull 2018;39:175–205.
4 Charrondiere UR, Stadlmayr B, Wijesinha-Bettoni R, Rittenschober D, Nowak V, Burlingame B: INFOODS contributions to fulfilling needs and meeting challenges concerning food composition databases. Procedia Food Sci 2013;2:35–45.
5 Finglas PM, Roe M, Pinchen H, Astley S: The contribution of food composition resources to nutrition science methodology. Nutr Bull 2017; 42:198–206.
6 FAO: Dietary Assessment: A Resource Guide to Method Selection and Application in Low Resource Settings. Rome, Food and Agriculture Organization of the United Nations, 2018. www.fao.org/publications.
7 Greenfield H, Southgate DAT: Food Composition Data: Production, Management and Use, ed 2. Rome, Springer US, 2003.
8 FAO: FAO/INFOODS e-Learning Course on Food Composition Data, 2013.
9 FAO/INFOODS: FAO/INFOODS Guidelines for Checking Food Composition Data Prior to the Publication of a User Table/Database – Version 1.0. Rome, FAO, 2012.
10 TBCA: Tabela Brasileira de Composição de Alimentos – Version 6.0. Univ São Paulo 406 (USP) Food Res Cent (FoRC), 2017. http://www.fcf.usp.br/tbca/ (cited April 20, 2018).
11 FAO/WHO: Human Vitamin and Mineral Requirements. Bangkok, 2001.
12 Toledo A, Burlingame B: Biodiversity and nutrition: a common path toward global food security and sustainable development. J Food Compos Anal 2006;19:477–483.
13 Rodriguez-Amaya DB, Kimura M, Godoy H, Amaya-Farfan J: Updated Brazilian database on food carotenoids: factors affecting carotenoid composition. J Food Compos Anal 2008;21:445–463.
14 Barata-Soares AD, Gomez MLPA, Mesquita CH de, Lajolo FM: Ascorbic acid biosynthesis: a precursor study on plants. Brazilian J Plant Physiol 2004;16:147–154.
15 Scheelbeek PFD, Bird FA, Tuomisto HL, et al: Effect of environmental changes on vegetable and legume yields and nutritional quality. Proc Natl Acad Sci U S A 2018;115:6804–6809.
16 Broberg CM, Högy P, Pleijel H: CO_2-induced changes in wheat grain composition: Meta-analysis and response functions. Agron 2017;7:1–18.
17 Thompson FE, Subar AF: Dietary Assessment Methodology; in Coulston AM, Boushey CJ, Ferruzzi MG, (eds): Nutrition in the Prevention and Treatment of Disease, ed 4., Academic Press, 2017, pp 5–48.
18 Global Fortification Data Exchange: Interactive Map, 2019. http://www.fortificationdata.org (cited April 20, 2019).
19 FAO: West Africa Food Composition Table, ed 2. Rome, Food and Agriculture Organization of the United Nations, 2012.
20 Grande F, Giuntini EB, Lajolo FM, de Menezes EW: How do calculation method and food data source affect estimates of vitamin A content in foods and dietary intake? J Food Compos Anal 2016;46:60–69.
21 INFOODS: International Network of Food Data Systems (website), 2018. http://www.fao.org/infoods/infoods/pt/ (cited February 8, 2019).

22 FAO/INFOODS: Food and Agriculture Organization of the United Nations. International Network of Food Data Systems. Food composition
challenges, 2017. http://www.fao.org/infoods/
infoods/food-composition-challenges [cited April
28, 2019).

23 Sivakumaran S, Huffman L, Sivakumaran S: The
New Zealand food composition database: a useful
tool for assessing New Zealanders' nutrient intake. Food Chem 2018;238:101–110.

24 Lopes T do VC, Giuntini EB, Lajolo FM, et al:
Compilation of mineral data: feasibility of updating the food composition database. J Food Compos Anal 2015;39:87–93.

25 Vila-Real C, Pimenta-Martins A, Gomes AM, et
al: How dietary intake has been assessed in African countries? A systematic review. Crit Rev
Food Sci Nutr 2018;58:1002–1022.

26 De Bruyn J, Ferguson E, Allman-Farinelli M, et
al: Food composition tables in resource-poor settings: exploring current limitations and opportunities, with a focus on animal-source foods in
sub-Saharan Africa. Br J Nutr 2016:1–11.

27 Longvah T, Ananthan R, Bhaskarachary K, Ven-
kaiah K: Indian Food Composition Tables. Hy-
derabad, National Institute of Nutrition. Indian
Council of Medical Research, 2017.

28 Charrondiere UR, Rittenschober D, Nowak V,
et al: FAO/INFOODS e-Learning Course on
Food Composition Data. Food Chem 2016;193:
6–11.

29 Schönfeldt HC, Hall N, Pretorius B: The important role of food composition in policies and programmes for better public health: a South African
case study. Food Chem 2018;238:94–100.

Michaelsen KF, Neufeld LM, Prentice AM (eds): Global Landscape of Nutrition Challenges in Infants and Children. Nestlé Nutr Inst Workshop Ser, vol 93, pp 51–62, (DOI: 10.1159/000503356)
Nestlé Nutrition Institute, Switzerland/S. Karger AG., Basel, © 2020

Balancing Safety and Potential for Impact in Universal Iron Interventions

Andrew J. Baldi[a] · Leila M. Larson[a, b] · Sant-Rayn Pasricha[a–e]

[a]Division of Population Health and Immunity, Walter and Eliza Hall Institute of Medical Research, Parkville, VIC, Australia; [b]Department of Medicine at the Peter Doherty Institute for Infection and Immunity, Parkville, VIC, Australia; [c]Department of Medical Biology, The University of Melbourne, Parkville, VIC, Australia; [d]Diagnostic Haematology, The Royal Melbourne Hospital, Parkville, VIC, Australia; [e]Clinical Haematology at The Peter MacCallum Cancer Centre and The Royal Melbourne Hospital, Parkville, VIC, Australia

Abstract

Almost 300 million children under 5 years of age are anemic worldwide. International policymakers recommend universal distribution of iron-based interventions – either iron supplements or iron-containing multiple micronutrient powders – to alleviate the burden of anemia in young children. When considering whether to implement universal iron interventions, it is essential to balance the putative benefits with possible risks. The key rationale for deploying universal iron interventions to reduce anemia in young children is to improve development, growth, and well-being. While plausible, few randomized controlled trials (RCTs) of iron interventions have carefully assessed these outcomes and there is currently inadequate evidence to support the hypothesis that universal iron interventions provide benefits on functional child health outcomes. Conversely, several important RCTs have found that when iron interventions are given to all children in a population, they may increase infection risk. Other possible risks of iron interventions have not yet been extensively described but include a risk of iron overdose and long-term iron loading in high-risk individuals. Identifying whether these interventions provide a net benefit or harm to populations is challenging. Until the quality of evidence for benefits improves, implementation of universal iron interventions in young children should be undertaken with caution.

© 2020 Nestlé Nutrition Institute, Switzerland/S. Karger AG, Basel

Introduction

Anemia represents a significant health burden globally. In its recent review, the World Health Organization (WHO) estimated that around 41% of children under 5 years of age were anemic worldwide in 2016 [1]. Anemia peaks in children under 2 years of age and generally improves as they reach pre-school age. In children, it is linked to rapid growth and increased demand for iron in erythropoiesis, as well as a potential reduction in iron intake due to reliance on complementary foods low in iron. Anemia risk is also influenced by factors including other micronutrient deficiencies, inflammation, infection, and the onset of disorders affecting red blood cell production or survival, such as hemoglobinopathies or thalassemia syndromes.

Iron interventions used to control anemia in large-scale programs in low- and middle-income countries (LMICs) may be given as iron salts (e.g., ferrous sulfate iron drops) but are increasingly being incorporated into multiple micronutrient powders (MNPs), which contain lipid microencapsulated iron (usually as ferrous fumarate or iron-EDTA) together with other micronutrients such as zinc, vitamin A, and ascorbate and enable home fortification of complementary foods.

The WHO recommends that such iron interventions be administered to all children in areas of high anemia prevalence [2, 3] (Table 1). The universal approach to iron interventions, using either iron drops or MNPs, is aimed at maximizing the benefits to children at a population level and avoiding the logistic and financial challenges of individual screening prior to supplementation. However, there is evidence of risk for young children, including significant associations with infection, and these must be included in the evaluation of these universal intervention programs.

This review will discuss some of the challenges relating to universal delivery of iron interventions, focusing on children under 2 years of age; it specifically does not pertain to clinical therapy for iron deficiency in diagnosed cases.

Determinants of Anemia

Anemia disproportionately affects children in LMICs in Asia and sub-Saharan Africa [4]. In these regions, there is an intersection between malnutrition, endemic infections including malaria, and genetic disorders of red cells, all of which contribute to the disease [5, 6] (Table 2).

Anemia has been previously proposed as a surrogate for low iron status in assessments of population nutrition status [7]; however, this fails to account for other causes of anemia and inevitably misses cases of iron deficiency in

Table 1. WHO guidelines for universal iron interventions in children aged 6–23 months [2, 3]

	Iron syrup/drops	Micronutrient powders containing iron
Iron dose	10–12.5 mg elemental iron	10–12.5 mg elemental iron
Intervention schedule	Daily for 3 consecutive months in a year	90 sachets or doses over 6 months
Target regions	Regions where anemia prevalence is 40% or higher*	Regions where anemia prevalence is 20% or higher*

Reprinted from WHO Guideline: Daily iron supplementation in infants and children, Table A, Page 2, Geneva: World Health Organization; 2016 and WHO guideline: Use of multiple micronutrient powders for point-of-use fortification of foods consumed by infants and young children aged 6–23 months and children aged 2–12 years, Table 1, Page 4, Geneva: World Health Organization; 2016.* From WHO guidelines: in malaria-endemic areas, these iron interventions should only be made together with "(public health) measures to prevent, diagnose, and treat malaria" [2, 3]. WHO, World Health Organization.

Table 2. Global prevalence of conditions known to contribute to anemia at the population level (excluding dietary iron deficiency)

Disorder	Prevalence in 2013 (all age groups) [5]	Prevalence of related anemia in 2013 (all age groups) [5]	Mechanism(s)
Malaria*	351 million	80 million	Multifactorial: intravascular hemolysis, chronic inflammation leading to reduced iron absorption/increased iron sequestration
Hookworm infection	472 million	35 million	Chronic blood loss
Thalassemias including thalassemia traits	208 million	105 million	Ineffective erythropoiesis
Sickle cell disease	3 million	3 million	Altered oxygen binding properties of hemoglobin S
G6PD deficiency	338 million	743,000	Intravascular hemolysis
Other micronutrient deficiency (folate, vitamin B12)	–	–	Reduced erythropoiesis
Anemia of inflammation	–	–	Reduced iron absorption and increased iron sequestration mediated by hepcidin

* 219 million cases in 2017 [6].
G6PD, glucose-6-phosphate dehydrogenase.

which the hemoglobin remains within the reference range [8]. Although iron deficiency has historically been considered the primary cause of anemia, accounting for 50% of cases [9], the WHO now estimates that 42% of cases of anemia in children globally can be corrected by iron supplementation, and in Africa, this figure falls to 32% due to the contribution by malaria [4]. The global estimated prevalence of iron deficiency among pre-school children is around 17% and of iron deficiency anemia is 10% [10]. It is thus almost certain that the contribution of iron deficiency to the overall prevalence of anemia is much lower than previously thought, making precise estimates difficult.

There are key limitations to assessing the true prevalence of iron deficiency and hence the number of children worldwide who would benefit from iron interventions. Given iron deficiency can exist separately to anemia and that iron deficiency can occur concurrent with other factors in an individual with anemia, devising population-level estimates of anemia determinants requires a sensitive and specific biomarker for iron status beyond relying on hemoglobin alone. Biomarkers for the estimation of iron status include ferritin, soluble transferrin receptor (sTfR), and hepcidin. Low ferritin is specific for iron deficiency and is commonly used in regions of the world where individual screening and treatment are employed. However, as ferritin is a positive acute-phase reactant, it may be elevated (or falsely normal) in inflammatory states [11]. Relying on hypoferritinemia alone for the diagnosis of iron deficiency, particularly in populations with a relatively high incidence of infection and inflammation, may underestimate true prevalence of iron deficiency. Furthermore, thresholds for defining iron deficiency remain uncertain, differ between different laboratories and expert agencies, and are not based on high-quality primary studies [12].

It may be feasible to use ferritin for population-level estimates of iron deficiency in areas of high infection prevalence by raising the usual cutoff level or correcting individual ferritin concentration for inflammation [11–13]. In an effort to account for inflammation, the Biomarkers Reflecting Inflammation and Nutritional Determinants of Anemia Project developed a model for interpreting serum ferritin concentrations in populations with inflammation, adjusting for inflammatory markers C-reactive protein and alpha 1-acid glycoprotein [14]. External validation of this approach is needed before this approach can be widely recommended. Implementation of direct iron status measurement for population estimates of iron deficiency will require utilization of a well-validated and reproducible approach that enables integration and adjustment of ferritin levels with inflammatory biomarkers and infection prevalence data.

Other biomarkers of iron status are available and may be useful in the future. The sTfR is raised in iron deficiency and is less influenced by inflammation, rendering it potentially more sensitive to iron deficiency [15]. However, its widespread implementation is limited due to several factors. First, it is also raised in increased erythropoiesis (e.g., hemolysis) and dyserythropoiesis (e.g., thalassemia syndromes) [16, 17], reducing its specificity [18]. Second, the assay is not commonly used, even in higher-income countries. Finally, there is variation between assays and therefore no standard reference range. Hepcidin is another promising biomarker of iron status. Studies in children have shown it to be diagnostic of iron deficiency, predictive of iron absorption, and capable of distinguishing anemia of inflammation from iron deficiency [19, 20]. However, like sTfR, hepcidin assays are largely ELISA-based and have substantial variation in values (although close correlation) between kits.

Even though researchers recognize the complexity of assessing iron deficiency, the case for screening of individuals is becoming more compelling. While WHO guidelines recommend universal intervention in areas of high prevalence, if only 30–40% of children are likely to respond and there are potential risks of delivering iron- to non-iron-deficient individuals, a more efficient approach may be to incorporate a more direct measure of iron status to screen at the level of the individual prior to administering iron. Individual screening, however, presents a significant logistical challenge, as iron measures need to be individually interpreted, and multiple encounters may be required for screening, commencing treatment, and evaluating response. Furthermore, given that the assays that most directly measure iron status are less widely available than other measures that use point-of-care instruments, their routine use would be problematic. Nevertheless, ambitious clinical trials are currently testing a "screen-and-treat" approach in the field and will provide important insights into the efficacy and feasibility of this method [21].

Due to the limitations of screen-and-treat approaches, iron interventions are universally distributed. It is therefore critical to define the net benefits and risks associated with universal iron interventions to justify this practice.

Evidence of Benefits from Universal Iron Interventions

Iron is an essential micronutrient required not only primarily for the synthesis of hemoglobin but also for other biological processes including neural development [22, 23]. Anemia, including iron deficiency anemia, has been associated in observational studies with adverse cognitive development in children and with reduced productivity in adults, resulting in significant economic consequences for LMICs [2].

Improvement of Anemia and Iron Deficiency

Iron supplementation improves anemia and iron deficiency. A systematic review and meta-analysis of randomized controlled trials (RCTs) found that daily iron reduced anemia by 39% and iron deficiency by 70% in children aged 4–23 months [24]. A similar review of MNP trials in young children showed a 31% reduction in anemia and a 51% reduction in iron deficiency [25].

Iron and Cognitive Development

There is limited quality evidence for functional benefits on child health from iron interventions. An important rationale for iron supplementation in infants and young children is to improve cognitive development. Observational studies consistently indicate that non-anemic children perform better on developmental assessments than their anemic peers [26]. However, few high-quality, double-blinded, well-powered RCTs exist that show benefits of iron supplementation on functional outcomes in children. Further, there is a lack of uniformity with regard to baseline population characteristics, iron dose, treatment age and duration, reporting of adherence to the iron intervention, and tools used to assess functional outcomes, particularly child development [23, 27, 28].

The most common developmental assessment tool used in iron trials is the Bayley Scales of Infant Development including the Mental Development Index (MDI) and the Psychomotor Development Index. Of the iron RCTs in children aged under 2 years living in settings with high prevalence of anemia, several show a modest benefit on child development. For example, Yousafzai et al. [29] showed that an "enhanced nutrition" intervention (MNP containing iron and other micronutrients) among 742 children aged 6–24 months was associated with higher MDI at 12 months and improved language at 12 and 24 months compared with the control group. However, as an effectiveness trial, this study was not placebo-controlled, and the intervention group received additional micronutrients aside from iron which likely contributed to the benefits observed [29]. An RCT in Indonesia randomized 680 infants aged 6 months to daily supplementation with iron, iron plus zinc, or placebo for 6 months. Following intervention, children in the iron group had significantly higher Psychomotor Development Index scores than did those in the placebo group. There were no significant differences in the other Bayley domains – including MDI – and the positive effect was not seen in the iron plus zinc group [30]. The lack of other evidence of positive effects on cognition may be in part due to many trials being underpowered to detect small changes on the assessment scales. A meta-analysis of children 4–23 months of age found no evidence of improvement in mental or psychomotor development scores following iron supplementation [24]. Current trials underway are recruiting larger cohorts with longer follow-up to better quantify the effects on cognitive development in children under 2 years of age [31].

Iron and Growth
Iron interventions do not benefit weight or linear growth in children in this age group [24, 25, 32]. Importantly, several trials have shown negative association between iron interventions and gains in weight and length [24]. Recent studies have found that more rapid child growth is associated with depletion of iron meaning children gaining the most weight have lower iron stores [33].

Evidence of Risk

While children in LMICs have a high theoretical potential to benefit from iron interventions, they also bear a large burden of infectious diseases including malaria, respiratory tract, and diarrheal infections.

Iron and Malaria
Malaria was estimated to be responsible for around 435,000 deaths worldwide in 2017 and 61% of these deaths were in children [6]. Endemic areas also show a high burden of anemia in addition to morbidity and mortality caused by *Plasmodium falciparum* malaria. In an anemic individual, iron supplementation, if effective, leads to a reticulocytosis, and these immature red blood cells are more prone to invasion by Plasmodium parasites [34]. An iron-deficient state appears relatively protective against malarial parasitemia and clinical infection [35].

The Pemba trial [36] was a major pediatric RCT of iron supplementation in a malaria-endemic region powered to assess adverse effects of universal intervention. It recruited 24,076 children aged 1–35 months from the Tanzanian island of Pemba and randomized children to receive one of iron and folic acid, iron and folic acid with zinc, or placebo. The 2 intervention arms containing iron were closed early due to an increased incidence of serious adverse events: a 12% increase in death or serious morbidity leading to hospital admission. Children in the iron-containing arms also had a 16% increased risk of serious adverse events due to clinical malaria compared to the placebo arm. The findings from this trial have had an ongoing impact on the landscape of global anemia control policy, prompting reconsideration of the universal intervention model as well as further study to determine how to deploy iron interventions safely in malaria-endemic areas [2, 3]. By contrast, a study of 1,958 children in

Ghana aged 6–35 months randomized to either an iron-containing MNP or an MNP without iron for 5 months showed no increase in malaria. These participants were given insecticide-treated bed nets at enrollment and cases of malaria were promptly treated [37]. There was, however, a 23% increased rate of hospital admission during the intervention period among those in the iron MNP group. Subsequent and current recommendations for children in malaria-endemic regions recognize the importance of the risks. A 2016 systematic review of 35 trials of iron interventions in children in malaria-endemic regions found that overall, iron interventions were not associated with increased clinical malaria. However, comparison between trials conducted in sites in which malaria prevention and management were present or absent showed that iron was associated with reduced clinical malaria where these facilities were present and with a higher risk of clinical malaria where they were absent, though quality of this evidence was evaluated as poor [38]. Recommendations from this review and from the WHO state that universal interventions should be implemented "in conjunction with public health measures to prevent, diagnose and treat malaria" [2, 3].

Iron and Diarrhea

Iron has been shown to reprofile the intestinal microbiota and increase markers of intestinal inflammation. Several studies of the intestinal microbiota in humans have shown an increased abundance of potentially pathogenic taxa and a reduction in commensal groups such as Bifidobacterium. This was evident in a study involving 2 RCTs of 115 six-month-old infants in Kenya receiving MNPs with and without iron. The infants who received iron had increased carriage of gut enteropathogens including Escherichia, Shigella, and Clostridium species. They also had significant increases in the intestinal inflammatory marker calprotectin by the end of the iron interventions [39].

Beyond changes in pathogen carriage and inflammation, large trials have also shown an increase in the incidence of diarrhea. A key study of 6-month-old infants conducted in Pakistan showed increased diarrhea with oral iron supplementation. These children were randomized to receive (1) an iron-containing MNP with zinc, (2) an iron-containing MNP without zinc, or (3) no intervention (control). Children in the arms receiving iron had a significantly increased proportion of days with diarrhea during the 12-month intervention, as well as increased bloody diarrhea [40]. A large non-placebo-controlled trial in Pakistan of iron-containing MNPs together with nutrition education and responsive stimulation showed a significantly higher maternal-reported diarrhea incidence in children who received iron compared to those who did not [29]. As these studies did not use a placebo, interpreting these adverse events must be done with caution.

Potentially pathogenic changes to the intestinal microbiota from iron may be influenced by the presence of environmental contaminants and therefore baseline pathogen carriage in the gut. Two similar iron intervention trials – one of children in Côte d'Ivoire and the other in South Africa – showed that higher enteropathogen carriage at baseline (Côte d'Ivoire) led to increases in these taxa at the end of the intervention, whereas in the South African cohort, there was lower enteropathogen abundance and no significant change with iron [41, 42]. There remains a paucity of evidence linking changes to the intestinal microbiota and the clinical outcome of diarrhea.

Iron and Respiratory Tract Infections
Iron supplementation has also been linked to respiratory tract infection. Soofi et al. [40] showed increased incidence of these infections among children receiving iron-containing MNPs. More recently, a double-blind RCT of 155 infants in Kenya showed a significantly higher incidence of treated respiratory tract infections in those receiving an iron-containing MNP (87%) versus those receiving no iron (75% – $p = 0.024\%$) [43]. However, the previously discussed meta-analysis of trials of children aged 4–23 months found no evidence of significant increase in the overall risk of acute respiratory infection or incidence of lower respiratory tract infection [24].

Risks in Iron-Replete Individuals
Additionally, the assumption that anemia is due to low iron stores fails to consider diseases causing anemia in which iron may not be required or is even contraindicated, such as thalassemia and hemoglobinopathies, which have high prevalence in several studies and whose distribution often corresponds to areas with current or previous malaria burden. For example, a case-control study in Mozambique performed thalassemia testing on participant samples and found an incidence of alpha thalassemia of 53% (including heterozygous and homozygous single-gene deletions). Participants with alpha thalassemia trait were overrepresented in anemic compared with non-anemic children [44].

Iron overload is a life-threatening disease that can lead to organ dysfunction including liver, heart, and endocrine failure [45]. While it is possible for children with thalassemia traits or syndromes to be iron deficient, in some conditions (e.g., HbE-beta thalassemia, beta thalassemia intermedia, hemoglobin H disease), there is a risk of iron overload brought about by ineffective hematopoiesis and increased intestinal iron absorption [46]. In South-East Asia, 2003 data showed that 44% of the population carried an alpha thalassemia mutation and there are also high rates of carriage of beta globin mutations and clinical syndromes of deletional and non-deletional HbH disease (such as hemoglobin H-Constant Spring) [47]. In the case of hemoglobin H-Constant Spring, iron overload can manifest in childhood [48].

Iron Toxicity

Finally, acute iron toxicity may result from ingestion of excess iron and lead to multiorgan dysfunction and, if severe and left untreated, death. This is a potential issue for programs that distribute iron in large quantities – for example, providing the total amount of iron syrup or tablets at a single initial time point – and where safety information is not provided to or understood by parents or guardians.

Conclusions

Anemia remains common in children living in LMICs. Universal iron intervention programs that aim to deliver iron to all members of a particular group assume that treating individuals with iron deficiency – and preventing iron deficiency in some of the others – makes this approach worthwhile. They also assume that the net benefit to the population is high because the benefits in the deficient group are high, the preventive effects in the non-deficient group are beneficial, and the possible risks in both deficient and non-deficient people are sufficiently low that supplementing them is inconsequential. While iron interventions in children have potential for enormous benefit, there is an urgent need to strengthen the evidence for the role of iron in improving child growth and development based on longer-term assessments and to clarify the risks associated with iron supplementation including infectious morbidity and risk of iron overload. Policymakers must consider risk-benefit when looking to open, continue, or expand universal iron intervention programs in children.

Acknowledgments

A.J.B. is supported by an Australian Government Research Training Program Scholarship provided by the Australian Commonwealth Government and the University of Melbourne. S.-R.P. is supported by an NHMRC Career Development Fellowship (GNT1158696) and NHMRC Project Grants (GNT1141185, GNT1159171, and GNT1159151).

Disclosure Statement

The authors have no conflicts of interest to disclose.

References

1　World Health Organization: Global Health Observatory Data Repository: Anaemia in Children <5 Years: Estimates by WHO Region, 2017.
2　World Health Organization: Daily Iron Supplementation in Infants and Children. Geneva, World Health Organization, 2016.
3　World Health Organization: WHO Guideline: Use of Multiple Micronutrient Powders for Point-of-Use Fortification of Foods Consumed by Infants and Young Children Aged 6–23 Months and Children Aged 2–12 Years. Geneva, World Health Organization, 2016.
4　World Health Organization: The Global Prevalence of Anaemia in 2011. Geneva, WHO, 2015.
5　Global Burden of Disease Study 2013 Collaborators: Global, regional, and national incidence, prevalence, and years lived with disability for 301 acute and chronic diseases and injuries in 188 countries, 1990–2013: a systematic analysis for the Global Burden of Disease Study 2013. Lancet 2015;386:743–800.
6　World Health Organization: World Malaria Report 2018. Geneva, World Health Organization, 2018.
7　World Health Organization: Iron Deficiency Anaemia: Assessment, Prevention and Control: A Guide for Programme Managers. Geneva, World Health Organization, 2011.
8　Joint World Health Organization/Centers for Disease Control and Prevention Technical Consultation on the Assessment of Iron Status at the Population Level: Assessing the iron status of populations: including literature reviews: report of a Joint World Health Organization/Centers for Disease Control and Prevention Technical Consultation on the Assessment of Iron Status at the Population Level. Geneva, World Health Organization, 2004.
9　de Benoist B, McLean E, Egli I, et al: Worldwide Prevalence of Anaemia 1993–2005: WHO Global Database on Anaemia, 2008.
10　Petry N, Olofin I, Hurrell RF, et al: The proportion of anemia associated with iron deficiency in low, medium, and high human development index countries: A systematic analysis of national surveys. Nutrients 2016;8:pii: E693.
11　Thurnham DI, McCabe LD, Haldar S, et al: Adjusting plasma ferritin concentrations to remove the effects of subclinical inflammation in the assessment of iron deficiency: a meta-analysis. Am J Clin Nutr 2010;92:546–555.
12　Daru J, Colman K, Stanworth SJ, et al: Serum ferritin as an indicator of iron status: what do we need to know? Am J Clin Nutr 2017;106(suppl 6): 1634s–1639s.
13　Garcia-Casal MN, Pena-Rosas JP, Pasricha SR: Rethinking ferritin cutoffs for iron deficiency and overload. Lancet Haematol 2014;1:e92–e94.
14　World Health Organization: Serum Ferritin Concentrations for the Assessment of iron Status and Iron Deficiency in Populations. Geneva, World Health Organization, 2011.
15　Beguin Y: Soluble transferrin receptor for the evaluation of erythropoiesis and iron status. Clin Chim Acta 2003;329:9–22.
16　Pasricha SR, Rooney P, Schneider H: Soluble transferrin receptor and depth of bone marrow suppression following high dose chemotherapy. Support Care Cancer 2009;17:847–850.
17　Jones E, Pasricha SR, Allen A, et al: Hepcidin is suppressed by erythropoiesis in hemoglobin E β-thalassemia and β-thalassemia trait. Blood 2015;125:873–880.
18　Feelders RA, Kuiper-Kramer EP, van Eijk HG: Structure, function and clinical significance of transferrin receptors. Clin Chem Lab Med 1999; 37:1–10.
19　Pasricha SR, Atkinson SH, Armitage AE, et al: Expression of the iron hormone hepcidin distinguishes different types of anemia in African children. Sci Transl Med 2014;6:235re3.
20　Bah A, Pasricha SR, Jallow MW, et al: Serum hepcidin concentrations decline during pregnancy and may identify iron deficiency: analysis of a longitudinal pregnancy cohort in the gambia. J Nutr 2017;147:1131–1137.
21　Bah A, Wegmuller R, Cerami C, et al: A double blind randomised controlled trial comparing standard dose of iron supplementation for pregnant women with two screen-and-treat approaches using hepcidin as a biomarker for ready and safe to receive iron. BMC Pregnancy Childbirth 2016;16:157.
22　Georgieff MK: The role of iron in neurodevelopment: Fetal iron deficiency and the developing hippocampus. Biochem Soc Trans 2008;36:1267–1271.
23　Larson LM, Phiri KS, Pasricha SR: Iron and cognitive development: what is the evidence? Ann Nutr Metab 2017;71(suppl 3):25–38.
24　Pasricha SR, Hayes E, Kalumba K, et al: Effect of daily iron supplementation on health in children aged 4–23 months: a systematic review and meta-analysis of randomised controlled trials. Lancet Glob Health 2013;1:e77–e86.
25　De-Regil LM, Suchdev PS, Vist GE, et al: Home fortification of foods with multiple micronutrient powders for health and nutrition in children under two years of age. Cochrane Database Syst Rev 2011;9:CD008959.
26　Grantham-McGregor S, Ani C: A review of studies on the effect of iron deficiency on cognitive development in children. J Nutr 2001;131(2S-2): 649S–666S; discussion 666S–668S.

27   Wang B, Zhan S, Gong T, et al: Iron therapy for improving psychomotor development and cognitive function in children under the age of three with iron deficiency anaemia. Cochrane Database Syst Rev 2013;6:CD001444.

28   Larson LM, Yousafzai AK: A meta-analysis of nutrition interventions on mental development of children under-two in low- and middle-income countries. Matern Child Nutr 2017;13.

29   Yousafzai AK, Rasheed MA, Rizvi A, et al: Effect of integrated responsive stimulation and nutrition interventions in the Lady Health Worker programme in Pakistan on child development, growth, and health outcomes: a cluster-randomised factorial effectiveness trial. Lancet 2014; 384:1282–1293.

30   Lind T, Lonnerdal B, Stenlund H, et al: A community-based randomized controlled trial of iron and zinc supplementation in Indonesian infants: effects on growth and development. Am J Clin Nutr 2004;80:729–736.

31   Hasan MI, Hossain SJ, Braat S, et al: Benefits and risks of Iron interventions in children (BRISC): protocol for a three-arm parallel-group randomised controlled field trial in Bangladesh. BMJ Open 2017;7:e018325.

32   Sachdev H, Gera T, Nestel P: Effect of iron supplementation on physical growth in children: systematic review of randomised controlled trials. Public Health Nutr 2006;9:904–920.

33   Armitage AE, Agbla SC, Betts M, et al: Rapid growth is a dominant predictor of hepcidin suppression and declining ferritin in Gambian infants. Haematologica 2019;104:1542–1553.

34   Clark MA, Goheen MM, Fulford A, et al: Host iron status and iron supplementation mediate susceptibility to erythrocytic stage Plasmodium falciparum. Nat Commun 2014;5:4446.

35   Gwamaka M, Kurtis JD, Sorensen BE, et al: Iron deficiency protects against severe Plasmodium falciparum malaria and death in young children. Clin Infect Dis 2012;54:1137–1144.

36   Sazawal S, Black RE, Ramsan M, et al: Effects of routine prophylactic supplementation with iron and folic acid on admission to hospital and mortality in preschool children in a high malaria transmission setting: community-based, randomised, placebo-controlled trial. Lancet 2006; 367:133–143.

37   Zlotkin S, Newton S, Aimone AM, et al: Effect of iron fortification on malaria incidence in infants and young children in Ghana: a randomized trial. JAMA 2013;310:938–947.

38   Neuberger A, Okebe J, Yahav D, et al: Oral iron supplements for children in malaria-endemic areas. Cochrane Database Syst Rev 2016; 2:CD006589.

39   Jaeggi T, Kortman GA, Moretti D, et al: Iron fortification adversely affects the gut microbiome, increases pathogen abundance and induces intestinal inflammation in Kenyan infants. Gut 2015; 64:731–742.

40   Soofi S, Cousens S, Iqbal SP, et al: Effect of provision of daily zinc and iron with several micronutrients on growth and morbidity among young children in Pakistan: a cluster-randomised trial. Lancet 2013;382:29–40.

41   Zimmermann MB, Chassard C, Rohner F, et al: The effects of iron fortification on the gut microbiota in African children: a randomized controlled trial in Cote d'Ivoire. Am J Clin Nutr 2010; 92:1406–1415.

42   Dostal A, Baumgartner J, Riesen N, et al: Effects of iron supplementation on dominant bacterial groups in the gut, faecal SCFA and gut inflammation: a randomised, placebo-controlled intervention trial in South African children. Br J Nutr 2014;112:547–556.

43   Paganini D, Uyoga MA, Kortman GA, et al: Prebiotic galacto-oligosaccharides mitigate the adverse effects of iron fortification on the gut microbiome: a randomised controlled study in Kenyan infants. Gut 2017;66:1956–1967.

44   Moraleda C, Aguilar R, Quinto L, et al: Anaemia in hospitalised preschool children from a rural area in Mozambique: a case control study in search for aetiological agents. BMC Pediatr 2017;17:63.

45   Fleming RE, Ponka P: Iron overload in human disease. N Engl J Med 2012;366:348–359.

46   Chui DH, Fucharoen S, Chan V: Hemoglobin H disease: not necessarily a benign disorder. Blood 2003;101:791–800.

47   Modell B, Darlison M: Global epidemiology of haemoglobin disorders and derived service indicators. Bull World Health Organ 2008;86:480–487.

48   Lal A, Goldrich ML, Haines DA, et al: Heterogeneity of hemoglobin H disease in childhood. N Engl J Med 2011;364:710–718.

Michaelsen KF, Neufeld LM, Prentice AM (eds): Global Landscape of Nutrition Challenges in
Infants and Children. Nestlé Nutr Inst Workshop Ser, vol 93, pp 63–65, (DOI: 10.1159/000503427)
Nestlé Nutrition Institute, Switzerland/S. Karger AG., Basel, © 2020

Summary on Pediatric Nutrition: Challenges and Approaches to Address Them

This session had the objective to provide an update on the global issues of malnutrition. The papers provide an up-to-date overview of the magnitude and distribution of malnutrition and focus in on what we know about what and how children are fed, including an in-depth review of the quality of dietary composition tables to permit such estimates. This was followed by a review of programmatic evidence of approaches to improving child nutrition, and the importance of considering both potential risks and benefits for iron interventions.

Progress toward eliminating all forms of malnutrition in children is lagging, and the global prevalence of stunting, wasting, overweight, and micronutrient malnutrition remains unacceptably high [1]. Childhood overweight is increasing in most regions, and with the limited data available, little progress has been made to addressing micronutrient malnutrition. Beyond simply tracking progress, a more profound understanding of the contextual etiology of the various forms of malnutrition and how this varies within and among countries is urgently needed to inform effective action.

What and how children are fed play a significant role not only in nutritional status but also in establishing healthy behaviors for optimal health, growth, and development [2]. International guidelines for feeding infants and toddlers exist including exclusive breastfeeding for 6 months, and complementary feeding with continued breastfeeding until 2 years of age. Caregivers' adherence to these guidelines, however, varies depending on the setting, access to information, quality of food, and cultural beliefs that often conflict with recommendations. Caregiver feeding style also plays an important role in what foods and drinks are offered and whether young children accept those foods. Feeding guidelines often include what is called "responsive feeding," which is the importance of caregiver attention to child cues of hunger and satiety. While there are data on food consumption and dietary diversity in early childhood, the literature on early childhood beverage consumption is limited. Such information is also of critical importance for the development of effective programmatic approaches that are responsive to local contextual realities.

Quantifying children's dietary intake is a key step in program design and critical for evaluating steps toward nutritional improvements. Accurate estimates of dietary intake in children and all ages requires food composition tables that are up-to-date and comprehensive of the types of foods included in the local diets, and the ways in which those foods may be prepared and consumed [3]. Despite food composition receiving more attention in recent years, many countries still need to generate and disseminate up-to-date and high-quality food composition tables and databases. Poor food composition data may lead to wrong conclusions resulting in the development of misleading policies and programs to improve the nutritional status of individuals and populations. This is particularly critical for micronutrients where the content may vary over time, with food processing (including fortification), handling, and cooking.

Several recent large-scale programs have aimed to improve child dietary intakes in low- and middle-income countries [4]. Programs have included behavior change techniques, provision of enabling social support, and/or adding objects to the environment such as food, supplements, or agricultural inputs or varying combination of these. The results of the programs have been mixed, with several showing important progress to addressing undernutrition but limited focus on overweight and obesity. Key success factors included the formation of alliances with key stakeholders, adequate financial and technical support, well-defined theories of change, and streamlined processes for monitoring and implementation. Factors that may limit success include poor quality/clarity of intervention design, inadequate utilization of behavioral theories or frameworks, insufficient adaptation to context, and several factors related to cost and feasibility.

Despite the promising results from several programs, some nutritional issues appear intractable [1]. Anemia, for example, remains common in children living in low- and middle-income countries, despite the existence of universal iron supplementation programs for children in many countries. Universal programs (i.e., those implemented without prior screening for anemia/iron deficiency) assume that the net benefit to the population is high because the benefits in the deficient group are high, the preventive effects in the nondeficient group are beneficial, and the possible risks in both deficient and nondeficient people are sufficiently low that supplementing them is inconsequential [5]. While iron interventions in children have potential for enormous benefit, there is an urgent need to strengthen the evidence for the role of iron in improving child growth and development based on longer term assessments and to clarify the risks associated with iron supplementation including infectious morbidity and risk of iron overload. Policymakers must consider risk–benefit when looking to open, continue, or expand universal iron intervention programs in children.

Lynnette M. Neufeld

References

1 Neufeld LM, Beal T, Larson LM, Cattaneo FD: Global landscape of malnutrition in infants and young children. In: Michaelsen KF, Neufeld LM, Prentice AM (eds): Global Landscape of Nutrition Challenges in Infants and Children. Nestlé Nutr Inst Workshop Ser. Basel, Karger, 2020, vol 93, pp 1–13.

2 Bentley ME, Nulty AK: When does it all begin: What, when, and how young children are fed. In: Michaelsen KF, Neufeld LM, Prentice AM (eds): Global Landscape of Nutrition Challenges in Infants and Children. Nestlé Nutr Inst Workshop Ser. Basel, Karger, 2020, vol 93, pp 15–24.

3 Grande F, Vincent A: The importance of food composition data for estimating micronutrient intake: what do we know now and into the future? In: Michaelsen KF, Neufeld LM, Prentice AM (eds): Global Landscape of Nutrition Challenges in Infants and Children. Nestlé Nutr Inst Workshop Ser. Basel, Karger, 2020, vol 93, pp 39–49.

4 Ramakrishnan U, Webb-Girard A: Improving children's diet: approach and progress. In: Michaelsen KF, Neufeld LM, Prentice AM (eds): Global Landscape of Nutrition Challenges in Infants and Children. Nestlé Nutr Inst Workshop Ser. Basel, Karger, 2020, vol 93, pp 25–37.

5 Baldi AJ, Larson LM, Pasricha SR: Balancing safety and potential for impact in universal iron interventions. In: Michaelsen KF, Neufeld LM, Prentice AM (eds): Global Landscape of Nutrition Challenges in Infants and Children. Nestlé Nutr Inst Workshop Ser. Basel, Karger, 2020, vol 93, pp 51–62.

Michaelsen KF, Neufeld LM, Prentice AM (eds): Global Landscape of Nutrition Challenges in Infants and Children. Nestlé Nutr Inst Workshop Ser, vol 93, pp 67–76, (DOI: 10.1159/000503359)
Nestlé Nutrition Institute, Switzerland/S. Karger AG., Basel, © 2020

Human Milk as the First Source of Micronutrients

Lindsay H. Allen[a, b] · Daniela Hampel[a, b]

[a]USDA, ARS Western Human Nutrition Research Center, Davis, CA, USA;
[b]Department of Nutrition, University of California, Davis, CA, USA

Abstract

Well-nourished mothers are assumed to produce adequate concentrations of nutrients in their milk for optimal infant growth and development and infants should be exclusively breastfed during the first 6 months. It is important to know the nutrient content of human milk as this information is used to set recommended adequate intakes (AIs) for infants. Our review of existing information reveals that the AI recommendations are based on poor data. The milk content of a few nutrients may not be adequate to provide requirements for 6 months even in well-nourished mothers. Importantly, the concentrations of many micronutrients in milk are low when the mother consumes a poor quality diet. Our new efficient methods for milk nutrient analysis have enabled us to illuminate the large differences in milk micronutrient concentrations across populations, to examine the effects of milk collection protocols on nutrient concentrations, and to study the effects of maternal supplementation in pregnancy and/or lactation on milk micronutrient and infant status. The ongoing Mothers, Infants and Lactation Quality study proposes to answer some of these uncertainties. Two hundred and fifty healthy, well-nourished, unsupplemented mother–infant dyads in each of the 4 countries are being studied. The range of milk nutrient concentrations across the first 9 months postpartum will provide "Reference Values" against which other studies and surveys can evaluate the quality of milk and possibly target nutrients for treatment with supplements or fortification.

Importance of Human Milk

Human milk is the best food for infants, especially during the first 6 months of life but continuing as an important supply of nutrients during the period of complementary feeding, which may last up to age 2–3 years [1]. Human milk contains immune factors that reduce the risk of infections; human milk oligosaccharides that support a healthy intestinal microbiome; and other bioactive factors with a range of beneficial functions. Breastfed infants have a lower risk of morbidity, mortality, and obesity and diabetes in later life and better cognitive development. Breastfeeding supports stronger mother-infant bonding; delays menstruation and subsequent conception; reduces risk of breast cancer; and is the most economical and environmentally friendly way to feed the infant. There are thousands of constituents in human milk that cannot be replicated in formula. Nevertheless, in this article we raise concerns about the adequacy of the micronutrient content of milk produced by women consuming poor quality diets and who could benefit from appropriate nutritional interventions. During lactation, women's requirements for most nutrients, including vitamins and minerals, are substantially higher than during pregnancy, to replace the amounts secreted in milk. The only nutrient for which the requirement is reduced is iron, due to cessation of menstruation.

Importance of Measuring Micronutrient Concentrations in Human Milk

Breast milk should be the sole source of all micronutrients during the first 6 months of life. The reported concentrations in human milk are used to set recommended adequate intakes (AIs) for infants; the accepted concentration of each nutrient (which we call the AI value) is multiplied by an assumed 780 mL/day intake of milk. The AI value is also used to estimate the micronutrient gaps that must be supplied by complementary foods. It is important to know the prevalence of low/inadequate milk micronutrient concentrations across populations. One way of estimating this prevalence is to express the actual concentrations in milk as a percentage of the AI values, an approach we use in this article. We need to know the effects of low milk micronutrient levels on infant status, growth, and development, but there is very little information on this important topic including the possible effects on early growth stunting. If milk micronutrient concentrations are low, there likely needs to be multiple micronutrient supplementation during pregnancy and/or lactation or improved dietary quality or fortification. Finally, for the many micronutrients in milk which respond to maternal status and intake, milk levels may turn out to be an efficient biomarker of population status.

Micronutrients That May Not Be Adequate in Breast Milk

For the first 6 months of life, breast milk definitely contains enough energy, protein, and fat and, in well-nourished women, enough of most micronutrients for optimal infant development. However, concentrations of iron, vitamin D, and iodine in areas of endemic iodine deficiency with inadequate universal salt iodization are likely to be inadequate to meet infants' requirements.

It is certain that iron concentrations in breast milk, which decline through the first 6 months, are not enough to maintain infant stores, but maternal iron supplementation during pregnancy or lactation does not increase the concentration in milk. Better strategies to improve infant iron status are to prevent anemia during pregnancy and delay cord clamping for at least 2 min after birth. WHO recommends that iron supplements (10–12.5 mg/day for 3 months a year) are needed by anemic infants aged 6–23 months and in areas where the prevalence of anemia is >40% and malaria prevention and treatment programs are available [2]. Low birth weight infants should be supplemented with iron after 2 months of age. There are potentially adverse effects of iron fortification and supplements on the intestinal microbiota that can increase risk of diarrhea in infants and young children [3].

Zinc concentrations in human milk also fall throughout the first 6 months of lactation and are below the AI value after about the first 5 weeks. This is to some extent an artifact of the milk concentration used to set the AI being the average concentration at 5 weeks. Moreover, zinc supplements for young infants are likely not useful in most situations [4], in part because the efficiency of absorption of zinc from human milk is high (>50%). In contrast, zinc supplements may be helpful for older breastfed infants with low zinc intake, low birth weight infants, and to replace losses resulting from persistent diarrhea [5].

Vitamin D deficiency, which will result in reduced deposition of calcium in infant bones, is relatively common globally, especially where exposure to sunlight is low, in persons with darker skin, and in urban areas with air pollution. Human milk is a poor source of vitamin D (<50 IU/L), and infants are born with low stores. Adequate infant status will depend on exposure of the infant's skin to sunlight and/or direct infant supplementation. The American Association for Pediatrics recommends infant supplementation starting soon after birth; 400 IU/day if breastfed. However, no supplement is needed if the infant is weaned to vitamin D-fortified formula, or to fortified milk after age 12 months, or if their face and hands are exposed to sunlight for a total of 2 h/week, or 30 min a week while wearing only a diaper. One attempt to increase the concentration of vitamin D in breast milk indicated that very high (6,400 IU/day) doses of vitamin D have to be given to the lactating mother [6] for the milk to supply enough of the vitamin to the infant so this is not common practice.

Iodine concentrations in breast milk need to be 100–200 µg/L to prevent deficiency in the infant. Breast milk iodine parallels maternal urinary iodine. An older review of 57 studies revealed iodine concentrations can be as low as 13–18 µg/L in women with goiter, 9–32 µg/L where the prevalence of goiter is high, and >90 µg/L where there is effective salt iodization. Insufficient milk iodine is common in areas of endemic iodine deficiency. WHO recommends giving 250 µg/day to lactating women in regions with moderate/severe iodine deficiency where iodized salt reaches <50% of households. In Morocco, 400 mg iodine given as oral iodized oil to the mother soon after delivery provided enough iodine to the infant for 6 months and was a more effective strategy than giving iodine to the infant directly [7]. In Switzerland, where mild to moderate iodine deficiency is prevalent, during the first year only infants predominantly fed with formula were iodine sufficient, based on their urinary iodine concentration [8] and even those fed complementary foods had poor status. Iodized salt may provide enough iodine for women and older children but infants consume very little salt.

There is no doubt that milk B12 falls substantially between about 1 and 6 months of life [9]. Scandinavian studies noted that infant plasma methylmalonic acid is highest around 6 months of age, when milk B12 is lowest, suggesting that B12 status is inadequate [10, 11]. This led to suggestions that maternal or infant supplementation may be necessary even in well-nourished populations [12]. However, there were no clinical signs of deficiency in these infants and such signs appear at much lower milk and infant serum B12 concentrations than in the Scandinavian studies [13].

Situations That Can Put Breastfed Infants at Risk of Micronutrient Deficiencies

The most common causes of micronutrient deficiencies in infant are summarized in Table 1. We have categorized micronutrients into 2 groups during lactation [14]. In Group I, milk concentrations are sensitive to maternal status and/or intake, so where the latter are poor the infant can become depleted (Table 2). Conversely, maternal supplementation can increase the micronutrients in milk. Nutrients in this group include most of the vitamins, iodine, and selenium. The milk concentration of Group II nutrients is independent of maternal status and/or intake, and increasing maternal intake has no effect on milk. These nutrients include folate, calcium, iron, copper, and zinc. Iron and folic acid supplementation during pregnancy is the standard of care in many locations, but these nutrients will not improve the quality of breast milk. In the opinion of these authors,

Table 1. Human milk micronutrients and their response to maternal status (updated from [16])

Group I	Group II
Milk MN $\propto$ to maternal status, infant depleted; supplements can ↑ MN in milk	Milk MN independent of maternal status, mother depleted; supplements have no effect on milk
B1, B2, B6, B12	Folate, calcium
Choline, vitamins A, D, E, K	Iron, copper, zinc
Iodine, selenium	

Table 2. Micronutrients and factors than can influence their concentrations in milk

Micronutrient	Situations that can put breastfed infants at risk of MN deficiency
Iron, vitamin D, iodine	Even milk of well-nourished women may not supply enough
Iron, vitamin A and B12	Low MN stores at birth due to poor maternal status in utero Preterm or low birth weight delivery – and higher postpartum requirements
All Group I MN	Low concentrations in milk because mother is deficient and/or has a low intake

securing adequate concentrations of all micronutrients in human milk should be a public health priority, supporting the argument for providing multiple micronutrients to pregnant women rather than iron and folic acid alone.

New Developments in Human Milk Micronutrient Research

In our laboratory, we have spent the last few years developing efficient, valid procedures for the analysis of micronutrients in the human milk matrix. These have been described in detail elsewhere [15–17] and rely substantially on liquid chromatographic techniques coupled with mass spectrometry for simultaneous analysis of multiple B-vitamins or fat-soluble vitamins. Vitamin B12 in human milk is bound to haptocorrin, which does not allow direct liquid chromatography-mass spectrometry (LC-MS) analysis, and has been shown to interfere with the analysis using competitive protein-binding assays, but solutions for its analysis in human milk have been described [18, 19].

We have also conducted a study in Bangladesh [20] that revealed that there is relatively little variation in milk vitamin concentrations in fore- versus hindmilk or due to diurnal variation and that the rate of appearance of nutrients from a micronutrient supplement provided to the mother varies greatly. A review of micronutrients in milk has been published including systematic reviews for vitamin B12, vitamin A, and iodine and a description of the analytical methods [21]. This work revealed that milk micronutrients have been measured in relatively few studies and that there are large differences in concentration in some of them (e.g., vitamin A and iodine) even among well-nourished women. There have been few longitudinal studies which is a major limitation since concentrations of most micronutrients change during lactation. The milk collection method, status, and diet of the mother and whether she has been supplemented are often not reported. Sometimes the analytical methods were invalid, especially for vitamin B12, riboflavin, iodine, and selenium. Our general conclusion is that some of the concentrations accepted for setting the AIs for infants and the additional requirements for lactation are questionable, and many of the recommendations relied on data from very few women [21].

As we have accumulated experience in measuring milk micronutrients, we have made many collaborations based on milk samples from around the world, some of them from micronutrient intervention trials, forming a picture of the large differences that exist among population groups. These results have been described in more detail elsewhere [22]. It is important to note that these samples were not nationally representative.

To summarize results for some vitamins, the global prevalence of thiamin deficiency is uncertain but the 2017 Cambodia National Survey found that 27% of women of reproductive age and 38% of infants aged 6–12 months were deficient [23]. Milk thiamin is sensitive to maternal status and increased on average from 29% of the AI value to 81% after Cambodian mothers were given high doses of the vitamin for 5 days [24] and from 66 to 100% of the AI when they were given fortified fish sauce during pregnancy and lactation for 6 months [25]. Our data show milk thiamin averaging 70% of the AI value in Cambodia and 50–60% in Ghana, India, The Gambia, Indonesia, and Peru. Older studies in Indonesia with beri-beri found that when concentrations were 60% of the AI, children grew slowly, and at 25% of the AI, they did not grow [26]. Other reported effects of thiamin deficiency include increased risk of mortality peaking around 3 months postpartum and retarded neurological and cognitive development, but the functional consequences of low milk thiamin remain to be determined.

The global prevalence of riboflavin deficiency is poorly documented but tends to be high in populations with a low intake of dairy products and eggs. In adults in the UK, Canada, Europe, and the Irish National Survey, 25–60% were depleted in the vitamin [27, 28]. Breast milk concentrations are affected rapidly by low maternal intake and increased by maternal supplementation. Our data show that levels are only 10–20% of the AI concentration in samples from Bangladesh, Kenya, Peru, Cambodia, Indonesia, and the Philippines. Severe deficiency causes growth retardation and developmental abnormalities in infants, but the effects of mild deficiency are not well understood.

Likewise, there are very few data on the prevalence of vitamin B6 deficiency. An older study showed abnormal infant behaviors associated with milk B6 <0.1 mg/L [29]. We found milk B6 to be <60% of the AI value in Cambodia, Bangladesh, rural Peru, Indonesia, the Philippines, Ghana, and The Gambia. Levels in Davis, California, were about 230% of the AI, likely due to the fact that ≈60% of prenatal supplements sold in the USA are high in this vitamin. Niacin can be synthesized from tryptophan, but it is possible that the infant uses more of this amino acid for protein synthesis. Status could be poor where maize is not treated with lime because its niacin is unavailable for absorption and where the diet is high in starchy foods and low in protein. We find very low milk concentrations in most countries, even in Davis, California, indicating that we know very little about true requirements for infants, which are likely overestimated.

More is known about the global prevalence of vitamin B12 deficiency, which is common across the life span in both males and females, due to inadequate consumption of animal source foods [30]. Breast milk B12 values track the usual intake of animal source foods, and the mother does not have to be a strict vegan to have low milk B12. We find very low milk concentrations in some countries, including Kenya, Guatemala, India, The Gambia, and Nepal. Dried fish and eggs may support more adequate milk B12 concentrations in some regions. The detrimental effects of B12 deficiency on infant development are well established as a result of clinical case studies of infants born to a mother with previously undiagnosed pernicious anemia or who is a vegan. There is a remarkable degree of growth stunting, small head circumference, and behavioral and other problems [13].

The infant's liver stores of vitamin A at birth are relatively small regardless of maternal status during pregnancy. Breast milk is a good source of the vitamin, and clinical deficiency symptoms rarely occur in breastfed infants during the first year of life. The normal milk retinol concentration is ≈485 µg/L and may fall to <300 µg/L in areas where maternal diets are low in vitamin A. Since infants need at least 300 µg/day to maintain their liver stores, many would become depleted when milk concentrations are low. Supplements provided to lactating mothers can provide their infants with a consistent and adequate supply of the vitamin in milk [31].

Effects of Maternal Supplementation on Vitamins in Human Milk

We have accumulated data from intervention studies in which micronutrients have been given to women during pregnancy and/or lactation, to determine if and when maternal supplementation is effective for increasing micronutrient

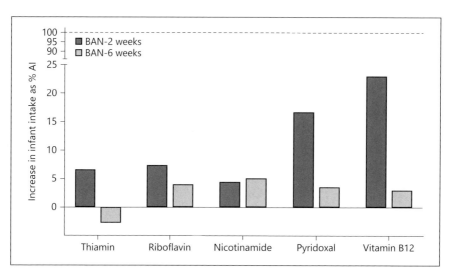

Fig. 1. Infant intake increase of vitamins through human milk at 2 and 6 weeks postpartum in the BAN study, expressed as % AI. AI, adequate intakes.

levels in milk. We have learned that only a small percentage of a dose given to the mother during lactation appears in milk. In the BAN study on exclusively breastfed infants in Malawi, daily supplements to the mother increased infant intake of the B vitamins by 5–23% of their AI at 2 weeks postpartum, but only by 0–5% at 6 weeks of age (Fig. 1) [32]. In the case of vitamin B12, a wide range of maternal doses given during pregnancy and/or lactation has had little effect on milk B12 content across countries. The main exception was in Bangladesh where 250 µg/day (10 times the Recommended Dietary Allowance) given from 20 weeks of pregnancy through 3 months postpartum increased milk B12 and maternal and infant status [33]. In Cameroon, providing the daily requirement for B12 by flour fortification did have an impressive effect on milk B12 concentrations [34]. A possible explanation is that when additional micronutrients are provided more than once a day in foods, then uptake by the mammary gland is more constant and milk concentrations are increased to a greater extent.

Establishing Reference Values for Micronutrients in Human Milk

We are currently establishing Reference Values for nutrients in human milk across the first 9 months postpartum. The Mothers, Infants and Lactation Quality study is enrolling 250 mother–infant dyads in 4 countries and collecting milk, and infant and maternal blood, 3 times during the first 8.5 months of lactation. The mothers are well nourished but not taking supplements or highly fortified foods. The Reference Values for nutrients in milk (a similar concept to reference values for growth) will enable more quantitative evaluation of milk quality within and among population groups and the need for and effect of interventions. AI values for infants will also be more accurate.

Acknowledgments

USDA is an equal opportunity employer and provider.

Disclosure Statement

The authors declare no conflict of interest.

References

1 World Health Organization: The Optimal Duration of Exclusive Breastfeeding. Report of an Expert Consultation. Geneva, World Health Organization, 2001.

2 World Health Organization: Daily Iron Supplementation in Infants and Children. Geneva, World Health Organization, 2016.

3 Paganini D, Zimmermann MB: The effects of iron fortification and supplementation on the gut microbiome and diarrhea in infants and children: a review. Am J Clin Nutr 2017;106(suppl 6):1688S–1693S.

4 Thomas TA: Zinc supplementation in diarrhea: summary of Cochrane database review. Curr Med Issue 2017;15:142–143.

5 Krebs NF: Update on zinc deficiency and excess in clinical pediatric practice. Ann Nutr Metab 2013;62:19–29.

6 Hollis BW, Wagner CL, Howard CR, et al: Maternal versus infant vitamin D supplementation during lactation: a randomized controlled trial. Pediatrics 2015;136:625–634.

7 Bouhouch RR, Bouhouch S, Cherkaoui M, et al: Direct iodine supplementation of infants versus supplementation of their breastfeeding mothers: a double-blind, randomised, placebo-controlled trial. Lancet Diabetes Endocrinol 2014;2:197–209.

8 Andersson M, Aeberli I, Wust N, et al: The Swiss iodized salt program provides adequate iodine for school children and pregnant women, but weaning infants not receiving iodine-containing complementary foods as well as their mothers are iodine deficient. J Clin Endocrinol Metab 2010; 95:5217–5224.

9 Dror DK, Allen LH: Vitamin B-12 in human milk: a systematic review. Adv Nutr 2018;9(suppl 1): 358S–366S.

10 Greibe E, Lildballe DL, Streym S, et al: Cobalamin and haptocorrin in human milk and cobalamin-related variables in mother and child: a 9-mo longitudinal study. Am J Clin Nutr 2013;98:389–395.

11 Hay G, Johnston C, Whitelaw A, et al: Folate and cobalamin status in relation to breastfeeding and weaning in healthy infants. Am J Clin Nutr 2008; 88:105–114.

12 Bjørke Monsen AL, Ueland PM: Homocysteine and methylmalonic acid in diagnosis and risk assessment from infancy to adolescence. Am J Clin Nutr 2003;78:7–21.

13 Dror DK, Allen LH: Effect of vitamin B12 deficiency on neurodevelopment in infants: current knowledge and possible mechanisms. Nutr Rev 2008;66:250–255.

14 Allen LH: Maternal micronutrient malnutrition: effects on breast milk and infant nutrition, and priorities for intervention. SCN News 1994;11: 21–24.

15 Hampel D, York ER, Allen LH: Ultra-performance liquid chromatography tandem mass-spectrometry (UPLC-MS/MS) for the rapid, simultaneous analysis of thiamin, riboflavin, flavin adenine dinucleotide, nicotinamide and pyridoxal in human milk. J Chromatogr B Analyt Technol Biomed Life Sci 2012;903:7–13.

16 Hampel D, Dror DK, Allen LH: Micronutrients in human milk: analytical methods. Adv Nutr 2018; 9(suppl 1):313S–331S.

17 Hampel D, Shahab-Ferdows S, Adair LS, et al: Thiamin and riboflavin in human milk: effects of lipid-based nutrient supplementation and stage of lactation on vitamer secretion and contributions to total vitamin content. PloS one 2016; 11:e0149479.

18 Lildballe DL, Hardlei TF, Allen LH, et al: High concentrations of haptocorrin interfere with routine measurement of cobalamins in human serum and milk. A problem and its solution. Clin Chem Lab Med 2009;47:182–187.

19 Hampel D, Shahab-Ferdows S, Domek JM, et al: Competitive chemiluminescent enzyme immunoassay for vitamin B12 analysis in human milk. Food Chem 2014;153:60–65.

20 Hampel D, Shahab-Ferdows S, Islam MM, et al: Vitamin concentrations in human milk vary with time within feed, circadian rhythm, and single-dose supplementation. J Nutr 2017;147:603–611.

21 Allen LH, Dror DK: Introduction to current knowledge on micronutrients in human milk: adequacy, analysis, and need for research. Adv Nutr 2018;9(suppl 1):275S–277S.

22 Allen LH, Hampel D: Water-soluble vitamins in human milk: factors affecting their concentration and their physiological significance; in Donovan SM, German JB, Lönnerdal B, Lucas A (eds): Human Milk: Composition, Clinical Benefits and Future Opportunities, Karger Publishers 2019;90: 69–81.

23 Whitfield KC, Smith G, Chamnan C, et al: High prevalence of thiamine (vitamin B1) deficiency in early childhood among a nationally representative sample of Cambodian women of childbearing age and their children. PLoS Negl Trop Dis 2017;11:e0005814.

24 Coats D, Frank EL, Reid JM, et al: Thiamine pharmacokinetics in Cambodian mothers and their breastfed infants. Am J Clin Nutr 2013;98:839–844.

25 Whitfield KC, Karakochuk CD, Kroeun H, et al: Perinatal consumption of thiamine-fortified fish sauce in rural Cambodia: a randomized clinical trial. JAMA Pediatr 2016;170: e162065.

26 Allen LH, Graham JM: Assuring micronutrient adequacy in the diets of young infants; in Delange FM, West KP (eds): Micronutrient Deficiencies in the First Months of Life. Nestec Ltd; Vevey/S. Basel, Karger AG, 2003, vol 52, pp 55–88.

27 Powers HJ, Hill MH, Mushtaq S, et al: Correcting a marginal riboflavin deficiency improves hematologic status in young women in the United Kingdom (RIBOFEM). Am J Clin Nutr 2011;93: 1274–1284.

28 Kehoe L, Walton J, Hopkins S, et al: Intake, status and dietary sources of riboflavin in a representative sample of Irish adults aged 18–90 years. Proc Nutr Soc 2018;77:E66.

29 McCullough AL, Kirksey A, Wachs TD: Vitamin B-6 status of Egyptian mothers: relation to infant behavior and maternal-infant interactions. Am J Clin Nutr 1990;51:1067–1074.

30 Allen LH, Miller JW, de Groot L, et al: Biomarkers of nutrition for development (BOND): vitamin B-12 review. J Nutr 2018;148(suppl 4): 1995S–2027S.

31 Dror DK, Allen LH: Retinol-to-fat ratio and retinol concentration in human milk show similar time trends and associations with maternal factors at the population level: a systematic review and meta-analysis. Adv Nutr 2018;9(suppl 1): 332S–346S.

32 Allen LH, Hampel D, Shahab-Ferdows S, et al: Antiretroviral therapy provided to HIV-infected Malawian women in a randomized trial diminishes the positive effects of lipid-based nutrient supplements on breast-milk B vitamins. Am J Clin Nutr 2015;102:1468–1474.

33 Siddiqua TJ, Ahmad SM, Ahsan KB, et al: Vitamin B12 supplementation during pregnancy and postpartum improves B12 status of both mothers and infants but vaccine response in mothers only: a randomized clinical trial in Bangladesh. Eur J Nutr 2016;55:281–293.

34 Engle-Stone R, Nankap M, Ndjebayi AO, et al: Iron, zinc, folate, and vitamin B-12 status increased among women and children in Yaoundé and Douala, Cameroon, 1 year after introducing fortified wheat flour. J Nutr 2017;147:1426–1436.

Michaelsen KF, Neufeld LM, Prentice AM (eds): Global Landscape of Nutrition Challenges in Infants and Children. Nestlé Nutr Inst Workshop Ser, vol 93, pp 77–90, (DOI: 10.1159/000503357)
Nestlé Nutrition Institute, Switzerland/S. Karger AG., Basel, © 2020

Role of Milk and Dairy Products in Growth of the Child

Benedikte Grenov · Anni Larnkjær · Christian Mølgaard · Kim F. Michaelsen

Department of Nutrition, Exercise and Sports, Faculty of Science, University of Copenhagen, Copenhagen, Denmark

Abstract

Cow's milk and dairy products intake increase linear growth in children and result in increased adult stature. This is supported by observational and intervention studies mainly from low- and middle-income countries. However, recent reviews primarily based on studies from well-nourished populations question the relation. The probable effects seem to be mediated by insulin-like growth factor-1 and insulin and to be more pronounced during periods of high growth velocity. Several components of cow's milk are suggested to stimulate growth: a high protein quality, bioavailable minerals that are important for growth, and perhaps lactose. Higher adult stature is associated with both positive and negative health effects. Growth stimulation is important in populations with undernutrition, but in well-nourished populations, it might not be important. A high intake of cow's milk and thereby a high protein intake early in life can increase the risk of later overweight and obesity, while a high protein intake later in childhood seems to be associated with a lower BMI later in childhood. A high dairy intake can limit the diversity of the diet and result in iron deficiency. Therefore, milk intake should not exceed 500 mL/day in young children. Most products for the treatment of undernutrition include dairy protein because of the well-documented effects on growth and recovery. However, as dairy is an expensive ingredient, the amount needed and the effects of alternative plant-based protein sources are considered.

Introduction

Milk has evolved as a food to support the offspring during a period of high growth velocity. Thus, it is not surprising that milk has specific growth-stimulating effects. This review focuses on cow's milk and as calves are growing at a very high rate, the content of protein and growth-related minerals is high in cow's milk. This has to be taken into account when giving cow's milk to young children that are growing at a lower rate. The purpose of the present review is to provide an update of the literature on cow's milk and dairy products on growth, with a special focus on linear growth and adult stature. The effects of milk intake on other aspects of growth, body composition, and risk of later overweight and obesity are also included. As there is consistent evidence that cow's milk intake has an effect on adult stature, a discussion of the complex association between adult stature and health outcomes is also included. Cow's milk has proven to be very effective in preventing and treating undernutrition, which will be discussed briefly. Throughout the review, the focus is on cow's milk given to children above 1 year.

Cow's Milk and Linear Growth

In a review published in 2006, we summarized the evidence of the effect of cow's milk on linear growth, based on studies from low- and high-income countries [1]. The review included the results of 6 intervention studies with milk to school-age children that showed an effect on height. The studies were from low-income countries, from the beginning of the last century, or included disadvantaged children, suggesting that the effect of milk was mainly seen among children who did not have an optimal nutritional status. The review also included several intervention studies in school children, which had no effect on height. The overall conclusion was that the strongest evidence that milk has an effect on linear growth comes from intervention and observational studies in low-income countries. However, observational studies from well-nourished populations in high-income countries also found an association between milk intake and linear growth, suggesting that milk has a growth-stimulating effect also when the nutrient intake is adequate. Since then many other studies, both observational and intervention studies and meta-analyses, some of which are discussed below, have supported that there is an effect of cow's milk on linear growth. This was also concluded in some recent reviews [2–4] but not all [15, 16].

Observational Studies

In a large cross-sectional study including data from 105 countries from Europe, Asia, North Africa, and Oceania, major correlates of adult male stature was explored [5]. Mean stature in the 105 countries was compared with the mean intake of 28 different protein sources based on national dietary data from FAOSTAT and 7 socioeconomic indicators. Among the protein sources, the strongest correlate was dairy protein intake ($r = 0.80$), while the correlation coefficient for meat protein intake was 0.67. As stature was also strongly correlated with many of the socioeconomic indicators, it is important to underline that this study is not proving causality, which is the case for all observational studies.

In a study from the US among girls aged >9 years all being premenarchal, dairy consumption was positively related to annual linear growth, peak growth velocity, and adult stature [6]. In one of their analyses, the association between dairy protein intake and annual height gain was equivalent to an increase of 0.9 mm per 10 g of dairy protein intake per day. Intake of nondairy animal protein and vegetable protein was not related to height or height velocity.

Wiley analyzed cross-sectional data from the NHANES study in the US and found that milk intake was associated with height in 12- to 18-year-old children, but not in 5- to 11-year-old children [7]. In a later analysis also from the NHANES study, it was found that in 2- to 5-year-old preschool children, those who were in the highest quartile of milk intake were significantly taller than the remaining children [8]. These data suggest that the effect of milk on linear growth is more pronounced during periods with high growth velocity.

In a study with 12,000 1-to 12-year-old children from 4 South East Asian countries (Indonesia, Malaysia, Thailand, and Vietnam), the association between dairy consumption and nutritional status was examined [9]. Dairy consumption was divided into 3 groups (<100, 100–199, and ≥200 mL), and the authors found significant lower percentages of stunted (HAZ ≤2) and underweight (WAZ ≤2) children in the high-intake group compared to the low-intake group, while there were no association regarding thinness (BAZ ≤2) and overweight (BAZ >2). These analyses were corrected for maternal education, income, and country. These 4 countries have high rates of lactose intolerance (primary lactase nonpersistence) [10], but the authors conclude that in young children this is not a problem and also that those with lactase deficiency can tolerate small amounts of milk and especially yoghurt, which has a lower content of lactose.

In a large cohort from the US with about 9,000 children, the association between milk intake at 4 years and height at 4 and 5 years was analyzed [11]. Those drinking more milk were taller at both 4 and 5 years, and the children drinking 4 servings/day (each 236 mL) were approximately 1 cm taller than those drinking <1 serving daily. In this study, there was also a positive association between milk intake and weight-for-height, which is discussed below under other growth outcomes.

In a longitudinal analysis of data from a cohort in the US, dietary intake and height were measured regularly between the ages of 2 and 17 years [12]. They found that the height of the children increased 0.39 cm for each additional 236 mL of milk consumed per day over the entire time span from 2 to 17 years. A strength of this observational study is the long follow-up period.

The Dutch are among the tallest in the world, and in a paper on the increasing secular trend in height, it was suggested that one of the explanations for the Dutch population being the tallest in the world could be a high consumption of dairy products, which is one of the highest in the world [13].

Intervention Studies

A systematic review and meta-analysis of 12 controlled interventions studies included studies from Europe, the US, China, Vietnam, Kenya, Indonesia, and India [14]. In 11 of the 12 studies, children were from 7 to 13 years old. The overall conclusion was that 245 mL of milk/day resulted in an increased linear growth of 0.4 cm/year. The effect was stronger in children with low height-for-age. Furthermore, the effect was strongest in teenagers, supporting that the effect of milk on linear growth is more pronounced during periods of rapid growth.

A recent meta-analysis of randomized controlled trials analyzed the effect of milk and milk product consumption on different aspects of growth in children and adolescents 6–18 years old [15]. Five of the 17 studies were also included in the review by de Beer et al. [14] mentioned above. The majority of the 17 studies included were from high-income Western countries. The studies were quite heterogeneous. A few older studies showing a positive effect on height were not included in the recent meta-analysis, and a number of newer studies that found either a negative or no effect of milk or milk product intake on height were included and the weight of each study differed between the 2 meta-analyses. In the recent meta-analysis, there were no effects on height (+0.09 cm, $p = 0.47$) or waist circumference or fat mass. However, there was a positive effect of milk and milk product intake on weight (+0.48 kg, $p = 0.001$) and lean mass (+0.21 kg, $p = 0.04$). The authors concluded that 6- to 18-year-old children consuming milk and dairy products are more likely to achieve a lean body phenotype. The reason there was no effect on height in this meta-analysis could be that the studies were mainly from high-income countries. A recent systematic review including many of the same randomized controlled trials as the 2 meta-analyses concluded that the effect of dairy product intake on linear growth is inconclusive [16].

Cow's Milk Allergy and Height
Several studies have shown that height is lower in children and adults with cow's milk allergy [17–19]. In these observational studies, there could be several reasons for the lower height. It could be lack of growth stimulation from milk. However, other factors associated with allergic diseases are likely also to influence growth. In a small study from Japan, they showed that children who were diagnosed with and treated for cow's milk allergy had an increase in height SD score during the year after they recovered and terminated milk avoidance [20]. In children with persistent milk allergy, there was no increase in height SD score.

Conclusion on Cow's Milk and Linear Growth
The large number of meta-analyses and observational studies supports that it is likely that there is an effect of milk intake on linear growth and adult stature, also in well-nourished populations. From the available studies, it is difficult to estimate the effect size of milk intake throughout childhood, but it is not likely to be more than a few centimeters or even less.

The Effects of Cow's Milk on Other Growth Outcomes

Several studies, reviews, and meta-analyses have examined the effect of milk intake on BMI, overweight, and obesity in children. A systematic review and meta-analysis of the long-term association between dairy consumption and risk of obesity included 10 studies with about 46,000 mainly school-age children [21]. The studies were mainly from the US and Western Europe and had an average follow-up of 3 years. Children in the highest intake group were less likely to be overweight or obese. For each dairy serving per day, the risk of overweight was reduced by 13% and the percentage of body fat was reduced by 0.65%.

In a study of >7,000 12-year-old children from Turkey, there was a significant negative association between milk intake and BMI [22]. This is in line with the meta-analysis of randomized studies by Kang et al. [15] mentioned above that showed an increase in lean mass and no significant change in fat mass, concluding that milk intake resulted in a lean body phenotype.

In an analysis of dairy consumption and cardiovascular risk factors in European adolescents, waist circumference and the sum of skinfolds were negatively associated with consumption of milk intake [23]. Another review concluded that the association between milk consumption and indicators of adiposity were neutral or negative [3].

However, other studies have found opposite associations. The study by DeBoer et al. [11] including 4-year-old children which found a positive association between milk intake and height also found that those with a high milk intake had higher risk of overweight and obesity. This is in line with another study from the US finding positive associations between milk intake and BMI [24]. The effect was stronger in the 2- to 4-year-old group compared to the 5- to 10-year-old group.

A reason for the conflicting results between milk intake and BMI could be different ages of the children included in the different studies. In younger children, a high protein intake has been associated with a higher risk of obesity, which is not the case later in childhood or in adults [25, 26].

An important aspect of growth, where there are convincing positive effects of cow's milk, is weight gain and recovery in children with moderate or severe acute malnutrition (SAM). Cow's milk components are essential ingredients in foods for treating SAM and are often used in foods for treating moderate acute malnutrition (MAM) [27–29]. The milk ingredients used in products for the prevention and treatment of MAM and SAM are typically dried skimmed milk (DSM) or whey protein. Whey has a specific effect on muscle protein synthesis if it is taken before or after exercise [30]. However, there is no evidence that whey has an advantage over DSM in the rehabilitation of undernourished children.

Another aspect of growth is bone health. In a recent review, the effects of milk and dairy products on bone health were discussed [4]. The authors concluded that there is an effect of milk on bone mineral content. However, they found that it is difficult to determine which components in milk cause such an effect. The content and bioavailability of calcium, high-quality proteins, vitamins (C, D, and K), and minerals (copper, manganese, and zinc) could all play a role. The effect of milk intake on bone mineral content was further supported by a recent systematic review of controlled trials [16]. They found that supplementing the usual diet with dairy products significantly increased bone mineral content during childhood.

Milk Intake and Age of Puberty
To understand the association between milk and dairy intake and adult stature, it is of interest to explore if there is an association between dairy intake and age at menarche. Women with early menarche have a shorter adult stature, which has been shown in both high- and low-income countries [31, 32]. As growth velocity after menarche is low, later menarche increases the period with higher growth velocity. However, this is not in accordance with the trend seen in countries where there is a secular increase in adult stature. In these countries, there has been a parallel decrease in age at menarche, indicating that other factors are influencing the association between timing of puberty and adult stature [32, 33].

In a study based on the large NHANES cohorts from the US, there was some evidence that a high milk intake was associated with a lower age at menarche and an increased risk of early menarche (<12 years) [34]. This finding was supported by a study from Iran in which they followed 4- to 12-year-old girls for a median of 6.5 years [35]. They found that the risk of early menarche was higher among those drinking more milk, after controlling for energy and protein intake. In a study from a slum area in India where age at menarche was high (mean 13.7 years), age at menarche was not associated with dairy intake [36]. Interestingly, a study from Chile found the opposite association. A higher intake of low-fat dairy products and yoghurt was positively associated with age at menarche [37].

In conclusion, several studies suggest that milk intake could have an influence on age at menarche, but the pattern is not clear. Nutritional status, habitual milk intake, socioeconomic status, or other confounders could influence the association.

Milk and IGF-I

Many studies and reviews have concluded that a higher intake of cow's milk results in an increase in insulin-like growth factor-1 (IGF-1) [1, 34, 38]. In a proof of concept study, we found that a very high intake of milk (1.5 L/day) for 1 week resulted in a significant increase in both IGF-I and insulin in 8-year-old boys, while there was no increase in IGF-I or insulin after intake of an equivalent, high amount of meat protein [39, 40]. To differentiate between the effect of casein and whey protein, we made an intervention study where 8-year-old boys received an amount of either casein or whey protein equivalent to the amount in 1.5 L of cow's milk [41]. The study showed that casein stimulated IGF-I and whey protein stimulated insulin, suggesting that one of the mechanisms behind the effect of milk on growth could be not only through a stimulation of IGF-I but also through a stimulation of insulin, which in children has a growth-stimulating effect.

In a cross-sectional study in India with 2-year-old children, there was a significant positive effect of milk intake (divided in 3 groups: <250, 250–500, >500 mL) on both IGF-I and length [34]. The same associations were seen in a Danish cohort study with 2.5-year-old healthy, well-nourished children, supporting that milk also has an effect in children with an adequate diet [42].

There seem to be a programming of the IGF-I axis, which has been discussed in detail in a review by Martin et al. [38]. Several studies suggest that a high intake of milk early in life results in higher IGF-I levels at this age but is associated with lower IGF-I level later in life. This indicates that the effect of a high milk intake early in life might be modified later, making the interpretation of the long-term effects of a high milk intake more complex. In one of our cohorts, we found a significant negative association between IGF-I at 9 months and at 17 years, supporting that there may be a programming effect [43]. However, the age at which the shift in IGF-1 level occurs is unclear.

Adult Stature and Health Outcomes

Since milk intake is associated with linear growth and adult stature, the association between adult stature and health outcomes is of interest. In populations where stunting is prevalent, there is no doubt that there are important negative outcomes associated with marked stunting like reduced cognitive function, shorter education, reduced work capacity and wages, and increased risk of disease [44, 45]. However, in populations where stunting is not prevalent, the consequences of differences of a few centimeters in adult high are complex. Many studies have examined the association between adult stature and noncommunicable diseases, and the overall conclusion is that adult stature is positively associated with the risk of cancer and negatively associated with the risk of cardiovascular diseases as outlined below, and it has been suggested that the IGF-I pathway has a central role in these associations [38, 46]. The associations with cancer and cardiovascular disease were confirmed in a large analysis of mortality due to chronic diseases from the US including almost 30,000 deaths [47]. Comparing the highest quintile of stature with the lowest, men had an 11% higher risk of dying from cancer and a 27% lower risk of dying from circulatory diseases. For women, the figures were 17% higher risk for cancer and 19% lower risk for circulatory diseases.

In an analysis of deaths among >1 million adults, followed for 16 million person-years, the effect of height on cause of mortality was analyzed [48]. Adult stature was inversely related to risk of death from coronary disease, heart failure, chronic obstructive pulmonary disease, and liver diseases but also some cancers (stomach and oral cancers). Being tall was positively associated with risk of death from pulmonary embolism, ruptured aortic aneurysms, and cancers of the pancreas, breast, ovary, prostate, colorectum, and skin (melanoma). The association between short height and coronary heart disease was also shown in a large meta-analysis including >3 million individuals [49]. They concluded that adults with the shortest stature category (<160.5 cm) had approximately 50% higher risk of coronary heart disease morbidity and mortality compared to the tallest stature category (>173.9 cm).

The association between adult stature and healthy aging was explored in a study based on the US Nurses Health study. About 50,000 women who had no chronic disease (e.g., cancer and type-2 diabetes) in 1980 were followed up in 2012 [50]. Healthy aging was defined as not having 11 major chronic diseases and no impairment of the memory, physical impairment, or mental health limitations. They found an 8% decrease in odds of a healthy aging for each SD increase in height. However, they also found that this effect was reduced in women with a prudent diet rich in vegetables and fruits.

In conclusion, the association between adult stature and health outcomes is complex. In populations where stunting is rare, being a few centimeters taller is not likely to have important overall beneficial or detrimental health effects. The few centimeters which a high milk intake may add are not likely to be important.

Growth Components in Cow's Milk
There are several components of cow's milk that are suggested to have a growth-stimulating effect [29]. The high protein quality score with a balanced content of specific amino acids is likely to play a key role. Furthermore, cow's milk has a high content of calcium and minerals important for growth such as potassium, phosphorus, magnesium, and zinc. The importance of a high protein quality in recovery from acute malnutrition was recently discussed in a review by Manary et al. [51]. They concluded that protein quality measured by the digestible indispensable amino acid score (DIAAS) had the strongest correlation with weight gain and that dairy protein, which has a high DIAAS score, was associated with better growth.

The effects of the high lactose content in milk on growth have been discussed, especially in relation to undernourished children [52]. Piglet studies have suggested that lactose can have a growth-stimulating effect compared to other carbohydrates, but this has not been shown in humans [52, 53]. The mechanisms behind such an effect could be a prebiotic effect on the microbiota and a positive effect on mineral absorption. However, secondary lactose intolerance can be a problem in some severely malnourished children, who can only tolerate reduced amounts of lactose during initial treatment. Regarding the effect of lactose in children from populations with a high prevalence of lactose intolerance (primary lactase nonpersistence), children rarely develop lactose intolerance before 3–4 years of age [10].

Potential Negative Effects of a High Milk Intake in Young Children
A high intake of cow's milk and dairy products in young children has potential negative effects [54]. This is potentially a problem in high- and middle-income countries where milk is easily available and affordable for many and where there is an awareness that milk intake may increase linear growth. A high intake of cow's milk results in a high protein intake, which can increase the risk of later overweight and obesity [25, 54–56]. Furthermore, a high dairy intake can limit the diversity of the diet. Iron deficiency can also be a problem because iron content is very low in cow's milk and because cow's milk has a negative effect on iron absorption. There is also a risk that a high intake of cow's milk from 12 to

24 months might replace breastmilk. This is mainly a risk in populations with a high prevalence of infectious diseases, as breastmilk also protects against infections during the second year of life [57].

Recommendations on Milk Intake
According to the WHO publication "Guiding principles for feeding non-breast-fed children 6–24 months of age," dairy products are needed if the infant is not breastfed [58]. If other animal source foods are eaten regularly, the recommendation is 200–400 mL of milk/day. If no other animal foods are eaten, the recommendation is an intake of 300–500 mL milk per day. Acceptable sources are full cream animal milk (cow, goat, sheep, buffalo), UHT milks, reconstituted evaporated milk or fermented milk, and yoghurt or equivalent amounts of milk powder added to complementary foods.

Some countries have recommendations for milk intake in children above 12 months that include an intake up to 750 mL. The government of Canada recommends an intake in 12- to 24-month-old children of 500 mL/day with an upper limit of 750 mL [59]. Centre of Disease Control in the US recommend 16–24 oz/day (470–710 mL) for children 12–24 months [60]. The recommendation in some South East Asian countries is 500–750 mL/day [9]. In a 12-month-old child, which typically weighs 10 kg, an intake of 750 mL whole cow's milk will cover about 55% of the energy intake, which will limit the diversity of the diet considerably. Furthermore, the protein intake from 750 mL of milk is about 2.5 g protein/day, more than twice the physiological requirement. In recommendations from Australia, an upper limit of 500 mL/day is recommended, and in Denmark, the recommendation for children above 12 months is about 350 mL with an upper limit of 500 mL [61].

Dairy ingredients are important in foods used to prevent and treat undernutrition because of the likely effects of milk on growth and due to the high quality of the protein. In a recent review, the specific guidance from UN organizations on the amount and source of protein for such foods has been summarized [27]. For therapeutic foods for the treatment of SAM in children below 5 years WHO, WFP and UNICEF jointly specifies that at least half of the protein should come from dairy ingredients. For ready-to-use-supplementary-foods used in the treatment of MAM, the World Food Programme specifies that at least 1/3 of the protein should come from DSM, whereas WHO only specifies that protein quality should be high. Specifically, the Protein Digestibility Corrected Amino Acid Score should be above 70%, which can be obtained through cereal/legume mixtures or milk or animal protein. The need for dairy protein in foods for MAM is discussed in a paper by Briend et al. [62]. As milk is an expensive ingredient, there is an interest in using lower quantities and to replace milk protein with high-quality plant proteins.

Conclusions

From the age of 1 year, cow's milk is an important part of a healthy diet providing important nutrients and supporting growth. There is some evidence that milk and dairy intake stimulate linear growth and increase adult stature. The strongest evidence comes from studies in low- and middle-income countries. However, a recent review and a meta-analysis, mainly based on studies from well-nourished populations in high-income countries, could not find a significant effect on linear growth. The mechanism seems to be mediated through stimulation of IGF-I and insulin secretion, and the effect may be strongest during periods of high growth velocity. The influence on adult height is not large, and increasing adult height in non-malnourished population seems to be associated with both positive and negative health implications. The overall pattern is that adult stature is inversely associated with the risk of cardiovascular diseases and positively associated with cancer risk.

A high milk intake in young children can have negative effects. The risk of overweight and obesity increases because of the high protein intake. In addition, a high milk intake will reduce the diversity of the diet and increase the risk of iron deficiency. Some authorities suggest an upper limit of 500 mL/day.

In populations with a high prevalence of undernutrition, the effect of milk and dairy products on growth, both linear growth and lean mass accretion, is important in preventing and treating wasting and stunting. UN organizations recommend dairy protein to be part of foods for treating SAM. A high milk content in foods for MAM makes it expensive, and the use of lower quantities of milk or using combinations of plant proteins with a high protein quality is considered.

Disclosure Statement

K.F.M., C.M., and B.G. have received unconditional research grants from USDEC, Arla, and Danish Dairy Research Foundation.

References

1 Hoppe C, Mølgaard C, Michaelsen KF: Cow's milk and linear growth in industrialized and developing countries. Annu Rev Nutr 2006;26:131–173.

2 Allen LH, Dror DK: Effects of animal source foods, with emphasis on milk, in the diet of children in low-income countries; in Clemens RA, Hernell O, Michaelsen KF (eds): Nestlé Nutrition Institute Workshop Series: Pediatric Program. Basel, KARGER, 2011, pp 113–130. https://www.karger.com/Article/FullText/325579 (cited March 12, 2019).

3 Dror DK, Allen LH: Dairy product intake in children and adolescents in developed countries: trends, nutritional contribution, and a review of association with health outcomes. Nutr Rev 2014; 72:68–81.

4 Yackobovitch-Gavan M, Phillip M, Gat-Yablonski G: How milk and its proteins affect growth, bone health, and weight. Horm Res Paediatr 2017;88: 63–69.

5 Grasgruber P, Sebera M, Hrazdíra E, et al: Major correlates of male height: a study of 105 countries. Econ Hum Biol 2016;21:172–195.

6 Berkey CS, Colditz GA, Rockett HR, et al: Dairy consumption and female height growth: Prospective cohort study. Cancer Epidemiol Biomarkers Prev 2009;18:1881–1887.

7 Wiley AS: Does milk make children grow? relationships between milk consumption and height in NHANES 1999–2002. Am J Hum Biol 2005;17:425–441.

8 Wiley AS: Consumption of milk, but not other dairy products, is associated with height among US preschool children in NHANES 1999–2002. Ann Hum Biol 2009;36:125–138.

9 Nguyen Bao KL, Sandjaja S, Poh BK, et al: The Consumption of Dairy and Its Association with Nutritional Status in the South East Asian Nutrition Surveys (SEANUTS). Nutrients 2018;10:pii:E759.

10 Itan Y, Jones BL, Ingram CJ, et al: A worldwide correlation of lactase persistence phenotype and genotypes. BMC Evol Biol 2010;10:36.

11 DeBoer MD, Agard HE, Scharf RJ: Milk intake, height and body mass index in preschool children. Arch Dis Child 2015;100:460–465.

12 Marshall TA, Curtis AM, Cavanaugh JE, et al: Higher longitudinal milk intakes are associated with increased height in a birth cohort followed for 17 years. J Nutr 2018;148:1144–1149.

13 Fredriks AM, van Buuren S, Burgmeijer RJ, et al: Continuing positive secular growth change in The Netherlands 1955–1997. Pediatr Res 2000;47:316–323.

14 de Beer H: Dairy products and physical stature: a systematic review and meta-analysis of controlled trials. Econ Hum Biol 2012;10:299–309.

15 Kang K, Sotunde OF, Weiler HA: Effects of milk and milk-product consumption on growth among children and adolescents aged 6–18 years: a meta-analysis of randomized controlled trials. Adv Nutr 2019;10:250–261.

16 de Lamas C, de Castro MJ, Gil-Campos M, et al: Effects of dairy product consumption on height and bone mineral content in children: a systematic review of controlled trials. Adv Nutr 2019;10(suppl_2):S88–S96.

17 Isolauri E, Sütas Y, Salo MK, et al: Elimination diet in cow's milk allergy: risk for impaired growth in young children. J Pediatr 1998;132:1004–1009.

18 Robbins KA, Wood RA, Keet CA: Milk allergy is associated with decreased growth in US children. J Allergy Clin Immunol 2014;134:1466–1468.e6.

19 Sinai T, Goldberg MR, Nachshon L, et al: Reduced final height and inadequate nutritional intake in cow's milk-allergic young adults. J Allergy Clin Immunol Pract 2019;7:509–515.

20 Yanagida N, Minoura T, Kitaoka S: Does terminating the avoidance of cow's milk lead to growth in height. EInt Arch Allergy Immunol 2015;168:56–60.

21 Lu L, Xun P, Wan Y, et al: Long-term association between dairy consumption and risk of childhood obesity: a systematic review and meta-analysis of prospective cohort studies. Eur J Clin Nutr 2016;70:414–423.

22 Koca T, Akcam M, Serdaroglu F, Dereci S: Breakfast habits, dairy product consumption, physical activity, and their associations with body mass index in children aged 6–18. Eur J Pediatr 2017;176:1251–1257.

23 Bel-Serrat S, Mouratidou T, Jiménez-Pavón D, et al: Is dairy consumption associated with low cardiovascular disease risk in European adolescents? Results from the HELENA Study. Pediatr Obes 2014;9:401–410.

24 Wiley AS: Dairy and milk consumption and child growth: is BMI involved? An analysis of NHANES 1999–2004. Am J Hum Biol 2010;22:517–525.

25 Hörnell A, Lagström H, Lande B, Thorsdottir I: Protein intake from 0 to 18 years of age and its relation to health: a systematic literature review for the 5th Nordic Nutrition Recommendations. Food Nutr Res 2013;57.

26 Thorning TK, Raben A, Tholstrup T, et al: Milk and dairy products: good or bad for human health? An assessment of the totality of scientific evidence. Food Nutr Res 2016;60:32527.

27 Caiafa K, Dewey KG, Michaelsen KF, et al: Food Aid for Nutrition: Narrative review of major research topics presented at a scientific symposium held October 21, 2017, at the 21st International Congress of Nutrition in Buenos Aires, Argentina. Food Nutr Bull 2019;40:111–123.

28 Grenov B, Friis H, Mølgaard C, Michaelsen KF: The role of human and other milks in preventing and treating undernutrition; In Nutrition and Health in a Developing World. New York, Springer Science + Business Media, 2017.

29 Grenov B, Michaelsen KF: Growth components of cow's milk: emphasis on effects in undernourished children. Food Nutr Bull 2018;39(2_suppl):S45–S53.

30 Graf S, Egert S, Heer M: Effects of whey protein supplements on metabolism: Evidence from human intervention studies. Curr Opin Clin Nutr Metab Care 2011;14:569–580.

31 Kang S, Kim YM, Lee JA, et al: Early menarche is a risk factor for short stature in young Korean females: an epidemiologic study. J Clin Res Pediatr Endocrinol 2019;11:234–239.

32 Onland-Moret NC, Peeters PH, van Gils CH, et al: Age at menarche in relation to adult height. Am J Epidemiol 2005;162:623–632.

33 Cole TJ: Secular trends in growth. Proc Nutr Soc 2000;59:317–324.

34 Wiley AS, Joshi SM, Lubree HG, et al: IGF-I and IGFBP-3 concentrations at 2 years: Associations with anthropometry and milk consumption in an Indian cohort. Eur J Clin Nutr 2018;72:564–571.

35 Ramezani Tehrani F, Moslehi N, Asghari G, et al: Intake of dairy products, calcium, magnesium, and phosphorus in childhood and age at menarche in the Tehran lipid and glucose study. PLoS One 2013;8:e57696.

36 Khopkar S, Kulathinal S, Virtanen SM, Säävälä M: Age at menarche and diet among adolescents in slums of Nashik, India. Int J Adolesc Med Health 2015 27:451–456.

37 Gaskins AJ, Pereira A, Quintiliano D, et al: Dairy intake in relation to breast and pubertal development in Chilean girls. Am J Clin Nutr 2017;105: 1166–1175.

38 Martin RM, Holly JMP, Gunnell D: Milk and linear growth: programming of the IGF-I axis and implication for health in adulthood; in Clemens RA, Hernell O, Michaelsen KF (eds): Nestlé Nutrition Institute Workshop Series: Pediatric Program. Basel, KARGER, 2011, pp 79–97. https://www.karger.com/Article/FullText/325577 (cited March 12, 2019).

39 Hoppe C, Mølgaard C, Juul A, Michaelsen KF: High intakes of skimmed milk, but not meat, increase serum IGF-I and IGFBP-3 in eight-year-old boys. Eur J Clin Nutr 2004;58:1211–1216.

40 Hoppe C, Mølgaard C, Vaag A, et al: High intakes of milk, but not meat, increase s-insulin and insulin resistance in 8-year-old boys. Eur J Clin Nutr 2005;59:393–398.

41 Hoppe C, Mølgaard C, Dalum C, et al: Differential effects of casein versus whey on fasting plasma levels of insulin, IGF-1 and IGF-1/IGFBP-3: Results from a randomized 7-day supplementation study in prepubertal boys. Eur J Clin Nutr 2009; 63:1076–1083.

42 Hoppe C, Udam TR, Lauritzen L, et al: Animal protein intake, serum insulin-like growth factor I, and growth in healthy 2.5-y-old Danish children. Am J Clin Nutr 2004;80:447–452.

43 Larnkjaer A, Ingstrup HK, Schack-Nielsen L, et al: Early programming of the IGF-I axis: Negative association between IGF-I in infancy and late adolescence in a 17-year longitudinal follow-up study of healthy subjects. Growth Horm IGF Res 2009;19:82–86.

44 McGovern ME, Krishna A, Aguayo VM, et al: A review of the evidence linking child stunting to economic outcomes. Int J Epidemiol 2017;46: 1171–1191.

45 Victora CG, Adair L, Fall C, et al: Maternal and child undernutrition: Consequences for adult health and human capital. Lancet 2008;371:340–357.

46 Stefan N, Häring HU, Hu FB, et al: Divergent associations of height with cardiometabolic disease and cancer: epidemiology, pathophysiology, and global implications. Lancet Diabetes Endocrinol 2016;4:457–467.

47 Sawada N, Wark PA, Merritt MA, et al: The association between adult attained height and sitting height with mortality in the European Prospective Investigation into Cancer and Nutrition (EPIC). PLoS One 2017;12:e0173117.

48 The Emerging Risk Factors Collaboration; Wormser D, Di Angelantonio E, Kaptoge S, et al: Adult height and the risk of cause-specific death and vascular morbidity in 1 million people: individual participant meta-analysis. Int J Epidemiol 2012;41:1419–1433.

49 Paajanen TA, Oksala NK, Kuukasjärvi P, Karhunen PJ: Short stature is associated with coronary heart disease: a systematic review of the literature and a meta-analysis. Eur Heart J 2010;31: 1802–1809.

50 Ma W, Hagan KA, Heianza Y, et al: Adult height, dietary patterns, and healthy aging. Am J Clin Nutr 2017;106:589–596.

51 Manary M, Callaghan M, Singh L, et al: Protein quality and growth in malnourished children. Food Nutr Bull 2016;37(1 suppl):S29–S36.

52 Grenov B, Briend A, Sangild PT, et al: Undernourished children and milk lactose. Food Nutr Bull 2016; 37:85–99.

53 Cromwell GL, Allee GL, Mahan DC: Assessment of lactose level in the mid- to late-nursery phase on performance of weanling pigs. J Anim Sci 2008;86:127–133.

54 Michaelsen KF, Grummer-Strawn L, Bégin F: Emerging issues in complementary feeding: global aspects. Matern Child Nutr 2017;13(suppl 2):e12444.

55 Michaelsen KF, Greer FR: Protein needs early in life and long-term health. Am J Clin Nutr 2014; 99:718S–722S.

56 Lind MV, Larnkjær A, Mølgaard C, et al: Dietary protein intake and quality in early life: impact on growth and obesity. Curr Opin Clin Nutr Metab Care 2017;20:71–76.

57 Victora CG, Bahl R, Barros AJ, et al: Breastfeeding in the 21st century: epidemiology, mechanisms, and lifelong effect. Lancet 2016;387:475–490.

58 World Health Organization: Guiding Principles for Feeding Non-Breastfed Children 6–24 Months of Age. Geneva, World Health Organization, 2005.

59 Government of Canada: Infant Nutrition Web-page. https://www.canada.ca/en/health-canada/services/infant-care/infant-nutrition.html (cited May 20, 2019).

60 Centers for Disease Control and Prevention. Fortified Cow's Milk and Milk Alternatives. https://www.cdc.gov/nutrition/infantandtoddlernutrition/foods-and-drinks/cows-milk-and-milk-alternatives.html (cited May 20, 2019).

61 Danish Health Authority: Ernæring til Spædbørn og Småbørn – en Håndbog for Sundhedspersonale (In Danish). https://www.sst.dk/da/Udgivelser/2019/Ernaering-til-spaedboern-og-smaaboern--en-haandbog-for-sundhedspersonale (cited May 20, 2019).

62 Briend A, Akomo P, Bahwere P, et al: Developing food supplements for moderately malnourished children: lessons learned from ready-to-use therapeutic foods. Food Nutr Bull 2015;36(1 suppl 1):S53–S58.

Michaelsen KF, Neufeld LM, Prentice AM (eds): Global Landscape of Nutrition Challenges in
Infants and Children. Nestlé Nutr Inst Workshop Ser, vol 93, pp 91–102, (DOI: 10.1159/000503358)
Nestlé Nutrition Institute, Switzerland/S. Karger AG., Basel, © 2020

Vitamin B12: An Intergenerational Story

Yajnik Chittaranjan

Kamalnayan Bajaj Diabetology Research Centre, Diabetes Unit, King Edward Memorial Hospital
Research Centre, Rasta Peth, Pune, India

Abstract

Vitamin B12 is a fascinating nutrient in that it is made by microbes but is essential for human
metabolism. Humans can get it only from animal origin foods. Dietary deficiency rather than
an absorption defect (Pernicious anemia, intrinsic factor defect) is the commonest cause of
deficiency in the world, contributed by cultural and economic imperatives. Indians have a
large prevalence of subclinical B12 deficiency due to vegetarianism. Birth cohort with long-
term serial follow-up (Pune Maternal Nutrition Study) has helped reveal the life-course evolution of B12 deficiency: genetics, transplacental and lactational transfer from the mother,
influence of family environment, rapid childhood and adolescent growth, and low consumption of milk all made a contribution. A novel association of low maternal B12 status was with
fetal growth restriction and increased risk factors of diabetes in the baby. After demonstrating adequate absorption of small (2 µg) dose of vitamin B12, and a noticeable improvement
of metabolic parameters in a pilot trial, we planned a supplementation trial in adolescents
to improve outcomes in their babies (a primordial prevention called Pune Rural Intervention
in the Young Adolescent). The results are awaited. The long-term effects in the babies born
in the trial will contribute to a better understanding of the Developmental Origins of Health
and Disease.   © 2020 Nestlé Nutrition Institute, Switzerland/S. Karger AG, Basel

Vitamin B12 is arguably the most fascinating of the nutrients. It is synthesized
only by prokaryotic microbes and thus contributed to the metabolism of the living
from early days of life on earth [1]. Its synthesis is complex and involves around
30 steps. Not all microbes are equipped to synthesize it and some are dependent

Table 1. Pernicious anemia versus nutritional deficiency

Characteristics	Pernicious anaemia	Nutrient deficiency of Vitamin B12
Eetiology	Genetic/autoimmunity Lack of intrinsic factor Defective absorption	Low dietary intake of Vitamin-B12, absorption normal Vegans/vegetarians Low socioeconomic status
Associated conditions	Autoimmune disorders (skin, thyroid, etc.)	Other nutritional deficiencies (Iron, folate, etc.)
Severity	Usually severe and symptomatic (Anemia, neurological and cognitive)	Usually less severe and asymptomatic
Treatment	Injectable, sublingual or high dose oral B12	Small oral doses effective

on an external supply. Vitamin B12-producing bacteria symbiont in some of the algae are an additional source of the vitamin [2]. Animals eat bacteria and their products and store vitamin B12 in their tissues; it enters the human food cycle when products of animal origin are eaten by the humans. The common nutritional source of the vitamin for humans is thus meat, liver, eggs, fish, and milk. Those who do not eat animal origin foods (due to ethical, religious, cultural, and socioeconomic reasons) are thus at a high risk of becoming deficient. Long-term use of drugs like metformin (for type 2 diabetes) and proton pump inhibitors (for acid peptic disease) and *H. pylori* infection also contribute to vitamin B12 deficiency by interfering different aspects of B12 absorption or metabolism.

Conventional Wisdom: Pernicious Anemia versus Nutrient Deficiency (Table 1)

The textbook description of vitamin B12 deficiency is usually based on the findings in cases of Pernicious Anemia, which is a genetically driven autoimmune condition [3]. It involves immune damage to the gastric mucosal parietal cells that synthesize the intrinsic factor. Lack of intrinsic factor stops vitamin B12 absorption from the gut and results in severe B12 deficiency. In addition to the direct effects of vitamin B12 deficiency (megaloblastic erythropoiesis manifesting as macrocytic anemia and subacute combined degeneration affecting spinal cord and peripheral nerves, dementia, etc.), there may be manifestations of autoimmune damage to other organs: hypothyroidism, type 1 diabetes, vitiligo, and so on. In the absence of intrinsic factor mechanism, treatment involves parenteral injections or high-dose oral (relying on absorption of vitamin

B12 by diffusion which is <1% of the dose) or sublingual (bypassing gastric-intestinal mechanisms) treatment. There is little information on lowest doses that are effective, and intuitively physicians consider large dose B12 treatment as safe.

There is now increasing recognition that a large proportion of vitamin B12 deficiency in the world is not related to intrinsic factor defect but to smaller intake of dietary vitamin. Vitamin B12 is present only in animal origin foods and some algae that harbor symbiotic B12-producing microbes. Plants do not have vitamin B12 as they do not require it. Reasons for vegetarianism and veganism differ in different populations. In a country like India, it is based on religious and cultural traditions (Jain, Hindu, and Buddha religions support vegetarianism), and it owes its origin to Samrat Ashoka (500 BC) who preached "ahimsa" (nonviolence) since he became Buddha's disciple. This suggests that vitamin B12 deficiency in these populations is multigenerational. In many parts of the world, poor socioeconomic conditions prevent purchase of animal origin foods and milk because they are expensive [4, 5].

Folate versus B12

It is also interesting to compare vitamin B12 and folate, the 2 vitamins with many actions in common because they both act on the same enzyme (methionine synthase which generates 1-C [methyl] groups which are crucial for multiple metabolic processes). Folate is of plant origin and, therefore, present in vegetarian foods. However, folate-rich vegetables and fruits can be expensive. Vitamin B12 has an additional influence on fatty acid and energy metabolism because it is also a co-factor for methyl-malonyl mutase enzyme which helps provide succinic acid and fatty acids for mitochondrial metabolism.

Folic Acid versus Folate

Naturally occurring folates are pteroyl polyglutamates, in reduced form and are damaged by cooking and exposure. On the other hand, the supplemental form folic acid is a synthetic monoglutamate in oxidized form that needs to be reduced in liver to active form. It is also heat stable, more bioavailable, and may circulate in free form in the absence of liver metabolism. Folic acid has a higher affinity for the folate receptor and could overstimulate the receptor or competitively inhibit natural folates from interacting with the receptor, with consequent ill effects.

B12 Studies in India

Our interest in vitamin B12 started when we serendipitously investigated homocysteine metabolism in our diabetic patients and nondiabetic controls in early 1990 in collaboration with Dr. Helga Refsum who visited Pune as a Rotary exchange fellow! She helped us make the measurements, and it was a surprise to find that 40-year-old Indians had twice the concentrations compared to Europeans. Interestingly, the difference was explained by high prevalence of vitamin B12 deficiency rather than folate deficiency, supported by elevated MMA concentrations. There was considerable resistance to acceptance of these data, despite previous publications [6, 7]. We investigated vitamin B12 status in urban and rural men in Pune [8], which confirmed the high prevalence of vitamin B12 deficiency and its strong association with hyperhomocysteinemia. This study revealed an interesting association: vitamin B12 deficiency was twice as common in the urban middle-class men compared to the slum dwellers and the rural men. This difference could be partly explained by the higher prevalence of vegetarianism, better education and hygiene, and higher obesity in the middle class. These associations were understandable because ultimate source of vitamin B12 in nature is microbes.

Equipped with this knowledge and possible role of 1-C metabolism in fetal growth and development, we investigated vitamin B12 status in pregnant women in the Pune Maternal Nutrition Study. This is a preconception birth cohort to investigate the role of maternal nutrition in fetal growth and its life-course risk of noncommunicable diseases. The mothers were young, short, and thin (21 years, 1.52 m, 18.1 kg/m^2) and ate mostly vegetarian diet of 1,800 cals/day (72% calories carbohydrates), 45 g/day proteins. The babies born were 2.7 kg and thin (ponderal index 24.1 kg/m^3). Interestingly, when compared with English babies (3.5 kg, 27.5 kg/m^3), they had thicker skinfolds for a given body weight, thus revealing the "thin-fat" phenotype of Indian babies. The food items that were strongly related to baby's size were those rich in micronutrients (green leafy vegetables, fruits, and milk). Further investigations revealed that maternal circulating folate concentrations directly associated with neonatal size, while homocysteine concentrations were inversely related. There was little folate deficiency in these mothers. Two of 3 mothers had low vitamin B12, 1/3rd had high homocysteine and 9/10th high MMA concentrations. High homocysteine concentrations predicted small for age indicating that deranged 1-C metabolism is associated with growth disturbance [9, 10].

When these children were followed-up, they maintained their thin-fat phenotype in relation to English babies into childhood [9]. We found that high maternal folate status during pregnancy predicted higher adiposity and higher insulin resistance in the children at 6 years of age (Fig. 1). Insulin resistance was the high-

Chittaranjan

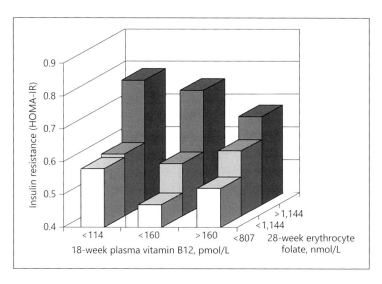

Fig. 1. HOMA-IR in the children in relation to maternal vitamin B12 (18 weeks) and red cell folate levels (28 weeks). Low maternal vitamin B12 (18 weeks) and high erythrocyte folate (28 weeks) predict high insulin resistance in the child at 6 years of age. Combined with the finding of higher adiposity in the children of mothers with high folate status suggests that maternal imbalance between these 2 vitamins during pregnancy may increase the risk of diabetes in the offspring. HOMA-IR, homeostasis model assessment of insulin resistance.

est in children of mothers who had low B12 but high folate status in pregnancy. Thus, an imbalance between vitamin B12 and folate status and the associated deranged 1-C metabolism appear to influence fetal growth, body composition, and future risk of diabetes ("programming") [10]. The high rates of vitamin B12 deficiency in this population favor a public health approach to improve the nutritional deficiency and influence intergenerational health in the population. Our further research therefore, included a formal test of vitamin B12 absorption and a pilot intervention with vitamin B12 to understand the size of the effect.

Vitamin B12 has the most amazing absorption and transport pathway, unmatched by any other nutrient (Fig. 2) [11]. In addition to that obtained from contaminant bacteria in water and food, dietary vitamin B12 is entirely from animal origin foods that is protein bound. This is dissociated from the protein in the stomach by the action of hydrochloric acid and binds to haptocorrin secreted in the saliva. This complex is further dissociated by the pancreatic and intestinal digestion, and the liberated vitamin B12 combines with intrinsic factor secreted by the parietal cells lining the stomach. This complex travels through the small intestine to the terminal ileum that has receptors for intrinsic factor (cubam) and is internalized in the enterocytes. It is transported across the intestinal wall by complex mechanisms and delivered to the transporting proteins in the circulation (haptocorrin and transcobalamin). The complex of vitamin B12

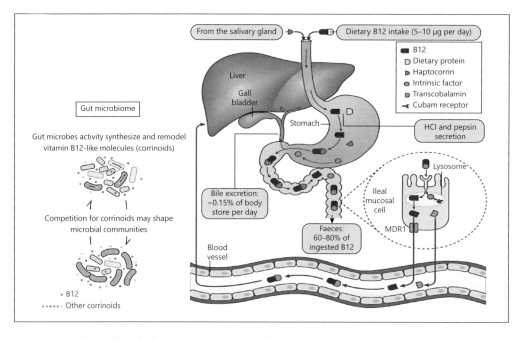

Fig. 2. Vitamin-B12 absorption. Vitamin B12 (B12) is mainly derived from animal sources. Following intake, it is released from its food carrier proteins by proteolysis in the acidic environment of the stomach, where it binds to haptocorrin. Haptocorrin is produced by the salivary glands and protects B12 from acid degradation. Degradation of haptocorrin and the pH change in the duodenum favour B12 binding to gastric intrinsic factor, which is produced by gastric parietal cells. The intrinsic factor-B12 complex binds to the cubam receptor (consisting of cubilin and amnionless). This receptor mediates the uptake of the intrinsic factor-B12 complex in the enterocytes of the distal ileum via receptor-mediated endocytosis. After lysosomal release, B12 exits via the basolateral membrane of the enterocyte, facilitated by multidrug resistance protein 1 (MDR1), and binds to transcobalamin, the blood carrier of B12 that is responsible for cellular delivery of B12. The majority of B12 is stored in the liver; some B12 is excreted in bile and undergoes enterohepatic circulation. A new consideration in the process is the role of the microbiome in B12 status of the humans. Microbes can both produce and utilize B12, and the composition of microbiome in the gut may influence host B12 status.

and transcobalamin II is called holo-transcobalamin and is the active form of circulating B12 that is taken up by receptors on the nucleated cells of the body. The complex with haptocorrin forms –70% of the circulating vitamin and is delivered to the liver where it is stored. Given the involvement of so many proteins (carriers) in the pathway of vitamin B12 absorption and transport, we would expect an association between the vitamin B12 status and genetics of the proteins that are involved. We performed a GWAS of vitamin B12 deficiency in our population and mostly found similar genetic associations as in the Europeans [12]. The genes involved in absorption pathway (TCN1, Cubilin, multidrug resistance protein 1, fucosyl transferase 2 [FUT2], and 6 [FUT6]) and transport

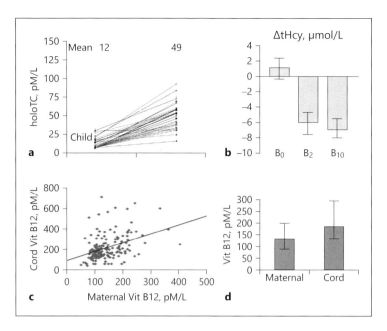

Fig. 3. Aspects of vitamin B12 metabolism in Indian children. **a** The rise in plasma holo-transcobalamin concentrations after 3 doses of 2 µg of vitamin B12 in children, suggestive of good absorption of oral low dose vitamin B12. **b** The substantial fall in plasma homocysteine concentrations in rural Indians after 1-year treatment with 2 and 10 µg/day. There was no significant difference in the 2 doses. **c** The direct association between maternal and cord blood B12 concentrations. **d** Stresses the point that cord blood concentrations are higher than those in the mother, suggesting active transport and storage.

pathway (TCN II) were associated. The strongest association worldwide is with a set of genes called FUT that are involved in posttranslational modification of proteins (fucosylation), which is an important requirement for "secretory" status and has been implicated in the gut-microbe interaction, which has substantial implications for the function of microbes in the intestinal wall. We found a novel SNP in FUT2 gene, and its specific role in B12 deficiency in Indians will be of interest. It will also be of interest to see if genetics will help tease out the role of maternal B12 deficiency in fetal programming of body composition and other systems that might increase future risk of diabetes.

We tested vitamin B12 absorption using the Danish protocol (Cobasorb) [13] (Fig. 3a). This involves 3 doses of oral vitamin B12 6 h apart and measuring circulating holo-TC concentration before and after. We used 10 µg tablet (as per protocol) as well as 2 µg and demonstrated that both doses were absorbed very satisfactorily. We then performed a 1-year pilot trial to test 0, 2, and 10 µg per day of vitamin B12 along with 0 or 200 µg per day of folic acid in a factorial design in 100 families (children and parents) [14] (Fig. 3b). The results showed that the B12 status improved after supplementation, 85% of the effect at 1 year was seen within 4 months. There was a 5 mmol/L decrease in circulating tHcy concentrations. Folic acid by itself had very little effect, and at these doses, we did not observe any side effects of either vitamin.

Daily requirements of vitamin B12 are around 2 µg, the ICMR in 2009 had suggested a value of 1 µg [15] (Narasinga Rao [15] 2010) which is lower than the NIH recommendation of 2.4 µg [16] (O'leary and Samman [16] 2010). We made a pragmatic decision to use 2 µg/day, avoiding larger doses because there could be metabolic adaptations in this population due to multigenerational nutrient deficiency and, therefore, protect against possible detrimental effects. Also, large doses would be unsustainable in public health because of the cost.

Our data from other studies showed a significant direct correlation between maternal and cord blood concentrations of vitamin B12, folate, and homocysteine [17] (Fig. 3c). The cord blood concentrations were higher than the maternal concentrations, indicating active transplacental transport and storage in the fetus (Fig. 3d). Interestingly, maternal vitamin B12 concentrations in pregnancy were still a significant determinant of child's B12 concentrations at 2 years [18, 19] and even 6 years of age. In addition, continued breast feeding at 2 years of age predicted lower and consumption of animal milk (cow or buffalo) a higher B12 status. These findings provided further support to improving maternal B12 status before, during and after pregnancy to benefit the child for its growth and development in utero as well as infancy. Equipped with all these results, we planned a vitamin B12 trial in adolescents in the Pune cohort to improve their nutrient status from before marriage and pregnancy with a view to improve the fetal growth and reduce the programming of future diabetes [20]. This would be a very substantial undertaking of time, effort, and money and involved cooperation from the participants. The final support for our decision came from the analysis (Mendelian Randomization) [9] of the maternal homocysteine-neonatal size association using maternal MTHFR C677T polymorphism as the genetic marker. The maternal T allele (rs1801133) was associated with elevated homocysteine levels and lower offspring birth weight (61 g, $p = 0.019$).

One of the interesting considerations in our research is the life-course trajectory of vitamin B12 deficiency in Indians and the possible contributions of various determinants. We have a unique opportunity to make such observations from the prospective birth cohorts in Pune (PMNS and the IAEA-B12 cohorts). The PMNS cohort was set up between 1993 and 1996 by enrolling the parents (F0), studying the pregnancies in F0 mothers, and serially following the F1 children as well as the parents for last 25 years. Interestingly, the F2 generation is now being born (many in the Pune Rural Intervention in the Young Adolescent trial), so we will be able to continue our intergenerational life-course story into the 3rd generation. In this article, we will discuss only broad observations because much of these data are being prepared for publication. On the other hand, the IAEA-B12 cohort has provided crucial information on maternal–offspring nutritional associations in early life.

In both the PMNS and the IAEA-B12 cohorts, we found a progressive fall in the circulating levels of B12 in the mother with advancing pregnancy. This has been described before and ascribed to fall in levels of haptocorrin that carries majority of the vitamin in circulation; levels of holo-TC remain fairly constant across gestation. There is a concomitant fall in circulating levels of homocysteine and albumin, suggesting a contribution of volume expansion and dilution of vascular compartment to the fall in the levels of different metabolites. Mother is the only source of vitamin B12 for the baby, and falling levels would also reflect active transfer across the placenta. Mother's vitamin B12 levels increased after delivery and then remained fairly constant in later years, as did in fathers. On the other hand, vitamin B12 concentrations progressively fell in the children (F1 generation) from childhood to early adulthood, accompanied by a progressive increase in homocysteine concentrations and the volume (MCV) of the red blood cells. Children have higher prevalence of vitamin B12 deficiency and hyperhomocysteinemia in late adolescence compared to their parents. The vitamin B12 status of the child is influenced by its genetics, maternal transfer during pregnancy and lactation, family environment (diet, hygiene, etc.), and growth during childhood and adolescence in addition to child's own dietary intake (especially of milk). This analysis helps to view vitamin B12 status in the "rainbow" framework in epidemiology, which highlights the interaction between individual's biology and "environmental" influences from family, community, and national and international ecosystems (Fig. 4). Religion, culture, and sociopolitical factors influence the phenotype through such ecosystems. Our model also resonates with the Developmental Origins of Health and Disease concept of evolution of health and disease in a life-course framework, with possible intergenerational and early life windows of opportunity for influencing outcomes (Fig. 5). On this background, it is obvious that cross-sectional associations, usually in the adults, will necessarily miss capturing the windows of opportunity for prevention.

Based on the findings in our various studies, we launched the Pune Rural Intervention in the Young Adolescent trial in 2012 under an Indo-UK research collaboration [21]. It involves the adolescent participants of the PMNS, starting at 17 years of age. We excluded those with very low vitamin B12 levels (<100 pM) in this placebo-controlled trial for ethical imperative and treated them with vitamin B12. The remaining participants were randomized to 2 µg B12/day as a capsule, with or without multi-micronutrients and the third arm is a placebo. All groups receive iron and folic acid tablets as per Government of India stan-

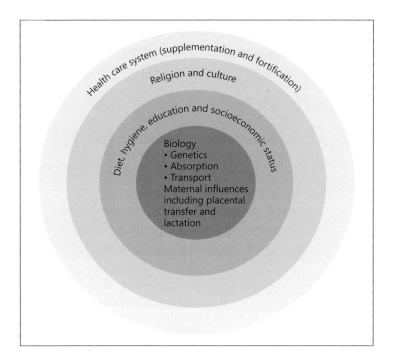

Fig. 4. Rainbow concept in the Epidemiology of vitamin B12 deficiency. Important factors that affect the demand and supply of vitamin B12 (B12) at the individual and population levels and throughout the patient's lifetime are highlighted. It is striking that the mother exerts a triple influence on the B12 status of the offspring: genetics, intrauterine and lactational B12 transfer, and postnatal family environment (socioeconomic status, hygiene, diet, religion, and culture). The father exerts a double influence: genetic and family environment. A female child will continue to propagate the direct maternal influences into the next generation. The suspected role of epigenetics in all 3 processes awaits elucidation. The nutritional status of the population and, therefore, the public health measures to improve it depend on the socioeconomic factors, religious and cultural practices, and the public health policies of the local, national, and international regulatory systems. Although targeting the B12 deficiency at an individual level is needed, more widespread interventions targeting the population are needed to influence prevalence of B12 deficiency in the population.

dards of practice. The ultimate outcome will be the diabetes risk in the children, but an interim outcome is the birth size and cord blood concentrations of vitamin B12 and multi-OMICs (DNA methylation, transcriptome, metabolome, proteome) in the cord blood. In addition, there will be a microbiome study of serial samples collected in the mothers and the children. The trial is ongoing, and due to socio-economic development and educational aspirations of the rural young, the rate of marriages is lower than predicted. Thus, at the end of 5 years of intervention, we stopped the trial in boys (only 21 marriages, 7 deliveries) but continued in the girls (over 150 marriages, 130 deliveries, 100 more expected in next few years). Even though we are blinded to the intervention groups,

Chittaranjan

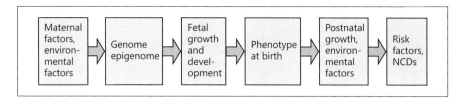

Fig. 5. Developmental Origins of Health and Disease describes the life-time evolution of health and disease susceptibility in an individual. On the background of the inherited "fixed" DNA sequence, chemical modifications in the genome regulate gene expression and therefore the phenotype of the individual. The most critical windows are in early life but continue to operate throughout the life (life-course model), manifesting in health and disease susceptibility.

we already have interesting observations on intergenerational changes in this rural population that is transitioning rapidly due to social and economic development. There is an increase in the height, BMI, and glucose and lipid concentrations of the pregnant daughters (F1 generation) compared to those in their mothers (F0), and their babies (F2) are bigger than their own size at birth.

Finally, we must discuss the exciting possibility that a part of vitamin B12 status of humans may be linked to the microbiome. Most of the thinking in this area is influenced by investigations of the gut (stool) microbiome. Only some microbes can synthesize vitamin B12 but not all of them [2]. Those who cannot, depend on external supply. Although classical thinking envisages bacterial colonization only in the distal colon, there is evidence for the presence of bacteria throughout the tract. A definite association of vitamin B12 deficiency is with *Helicobacter pylori* infection in the stomach [22]. This may be due to chronic gastritis that affects the production of acid and intrinsic factor. Stool microbiome studies have mostly shown an association between over population of vitamin B12 requiring bacteria rather than a paucity of B12-producing bacteria [2]. Some probiotics have caused a small increase in vitamin B12 status. Further studies are needed to expand the microbiome story for vitamin B12 nutrition, including intergenerational transfer from the mother to the baby. It will be important to study these issues in Indians who have a different microbiome compared to Europeans.

Acknowledgments

Dr. Krishna Sukla and Sonali Wagle helped in the organization of this article. Dr. Yajnik has been funded by The Wellcome Trust, London, UK, The MRC, UK, The Nestle Foundation, Switzerland, The Department of Biotechnology, Govt. of India, Indian Council of Medical Research, and The International Atomic Energy Agency, Vienna, for different studies which contributed the data used for this article.

Disclosure Statement

The author declares no conflicts of interest in relation to this article.

References

1 Martens JH, Barg H, Warren MJ, et al: Microbial production of vitamin B12. Appl Microbiol Biotechnol 2002;58:275–285.
2 Degnan PH, Taga ME, Goodman AL: Vitamin B12 as a modulator of gut microbial ecology. Cell Metab 2014;20:769–778.
3 Banka S, Ryan K, Thomson W, et al: Pernicious anemia – genetic insights. Autoimmun Rev 2011; 10:455–459.
4 Allen LH: Folate and vitamin B12 status in the Americas. Nutr Rev 2004;62:S29–S33.
5 Allen LH: How common is vitamin B-12 deficiency? Am J Clin Nutr 2009;89:S693–S696.
6 Chanarin I, Malkowska V, O'Hea AM, et al: Megaloblastic anaemia in a vegetarian Hindu community. Lancet 1985;2:1168–1172.
7 Mathan VI: Tropical sprue in Southern India. Trans R Soc Trop Med Hyg 1988;82:10–14.
8 Yajnik CS, Deshpande SS, Lubree HG, et al: Vitamin B12 deficiency and hyperhomocysteinemia in rural and urban Indians. J Assoc Physicians India 2006;54:775–782.
9 Yajnik CS, Chandak GR, Joglekar C, et al: Maternal homocysteine in pregnancy and offspring birthweight: epidemiological associations and Mendelian randomization analysis. Int J Epidemiol 2014;43:e1487–e1497.
10 Yajnik CS, Deshpande SS, Jackson AA, et al: Vitamin B12 and folate concentrations during pregnancy and insulin resistance in the offspring: the Pune Maternal Nutrition Study. Diabetologia 2008;51:29–38.
11 Green R, Allen LH, Bjorke-Monsen A, et al: Vitamin B12 deficiency. Nat Rev Dis Primers 2017;3: 17040.
12 Nongmaithem SS, Joglekar CV, Krishnaveni GV, et al: GWAS identifies population-specific new regulatory variants in FUT6 associated with plasma B12 concentrations in Indians. Hum Mol Genet 2017;26:2589.
13 Bhat DS, Thuse NV, Lubree HG, et al: Increases in plasma holotranscobalamin can be used to assess vitamin B-12 absorption in individuals with low plasma vitamin B-12. J Nutr 2009;139: 2119–2123.
14 Deshmukh US, Joglekar CV, Lubree HG, et al: Effect of physiological doses of oral vitamin b12 on plasma homocysteine: A randomized, placebo-controlled, double-blind trial in india. Eur J Clin Nutr 2010;64:495–502.
15 Narasinga Rao BS: Nutrient requirement and safe dietary intake for Indians. NFI Bull 2010;31:1–8.
16 O'Leary F, Samman S: Vitamin B12 in health and disease. Nutrients 2010;2:299–316.
17 Yajnik CS, Deshmukh US: Fetal programming: maternal nutrition and role of one-carbon metabolism. Rev Endocr Metab Disord 2012;13: 121–127.
18 Lubree HG, Katre PA, Joshi SM, et al: Child's homocysteine concentration at 2 years is influenced by pregnancy vitamin B12 and folate status. J Dev Orig Health Dis 2012;3:32–38.
19 Bhate VK, Joshi SM, Ladkat RS, et al: Vitamin B12 and folate during pregnancy and offspring motor, mental and social development at 2 years of age. J Dev Orig Health Dis 2012;3:123–130.
20 Saravanan P, Yajnik CS: Role of maternal vitamin B12 on the metabolic health of the offspring: a contributor to the diabetes epidemic? Br J Diabetes Vasc Dis 2010;10:109–114.
21 Kumaran K, Yajnik P, Lubree H, et al: The Pune Rural Intervention in Young Adolescents (PRIYA) study: design and methods. BMC Nutrition 2017;3:41.
22 Kaptan K, Beyan C, Ural AU, et al: Helicobacter pylori – is it a novel causative agent in Vitamin B12 deficiency? Arch Intern Med 2000;160:1349–1353.

Michaelsen KF, Neufeld LM, Prentice AM (eds): Global Landscape of Nutrition Challenges in
Infants and Children. Nestlé Nutr Inst Workshop Ser, vol 93, pp 103–110, (DOI: 10.1159/000503348)
Nestlé Nutrition Institute, Switzerland/S. Karger AG., Basel, © 2020

Vegan Diet in Young Children

Pascal Müller

Children's Hospital of Eastern Switzerland, St. Gallen, Switzerland

Abstract

The prevalence of restrictive diets, mainly vegetarian and vegan, is markedly on the increase in Europe and other Western countries. In young children and adolescents, not only weight and height but also neurocognitive and psychomotor development are all strongly influenced by the source, quantity, and quality of their nutrition. In studies done mainly in adult populations, a plant-based diet showed benefits in the reduced risk of chronic diseases such as obesity, type 2 diabetes, cardiovascular diseases, and some types of cancer. However, there is no clear evidence that a vegan diet started in early childhood confers a lasting health benefit. On the other hand, a vegan diet can be potentially critical for young children with risks of inadequate supply in terms of protein quality and energy as well as long-chain fatty acids, iron, zinc, vitamin D, iodine, calcium, and particularly vitamin B12. Deficiencies in these nutrients can lead to severe and sometimes irreversible developmental disorders. If such a diet is chosen for ethical, ecological, or health reasons, a well-planned, diversified diet with additional supplementation of vitamin B12, vitamin D, iodine, and potentially other micronutrients is crucial to ensure a healthy and nutritious intake during childhood.

© 2020 Nestlé Nutrition Institute, Switzerland/S. Karger AG, Basel

In addition to regions where vegetarian and vegan diets have a long cultural- and religious-based tradition, these diets have recently become more and more prevalent in Europe and other Western countries. It is estimated that the prevalence of vegan adolescents and adults in Western Europe countries ranges from around 0.2 to 3% [1]. Reliable population-based numbers on vegan-fed infants and young chil-

Table 1. Definitions of vegetarian and vegan diets, adapted from [1]

Type of diet (selection, preparation)	Summary of definitions collected from numerous sources, abridged
Flexitarian (semi-vegetarian)/ meat reductionism/ reducetarian	Occasional inclusion (less than once per week) of flesh foodstuff (meat, poultry, and fish) and permits eating all other animal products (e.g., eggs, milk, honey)
General vegetarian diets	Whenever not specified, a vegetarian diet is often an ovo-lacto-vegetarian diet
Pescetarian (pesco-vegetarian)	Includes seafood/fish, but not flesh of other animals (meat, poultry), and permits eating all other animal products (e.g., eggs, milk, honey). This diet is sometimes included in the semi-vegetarian group
Pollo-vegetarian	Poultry is the only animal flesh consumed, as well as dairy and egg products. This diet is sometimes included in the semi-vegetarian group
Ovo-lacto-vegetarian	Excludes all types of flesh foodstuffs (meat, poultry, fish), but permits eating all other animal products (e.g., eggs, milk, honey)
Lacto-vegetarian	Excludes flesh foodstuffs and eggs but allows dairy products, honey
Ovo-vegetarian	Excludes consumption of all animal products with the exception of eggs
Vegan	Diet which excludes all animal products (both as ingredients and processing aids, the latter being an important aspect); an exception is human mother's breast milk, given voluntarily; veganism can also imply excluding all items of animal origin (e.g., made from wool, silk, leather materials) Other subcategories of a vegan diet are: – *Vitarian (raw vegan):* Permits consumption of organic, raw, and fresh foods only; excludes coffee and tea – *Fruitarian:* Excludes flesh foodstuffs, animal products, and vegetables, cereals → permitted are only fruit, nuts, seeds, which can be gathered without damaging the plant – *Sproutarian:* Eating foods in the form of sprouted plant seedlings, such as grains, vegetables, fruits

dren are not available. Furthermore, little is known about the duration of a vegan diet in this population group. A recent survey in Switzerland found that a majority of vegans (76%) had followed a vegan diet for <5 years [2] and only 2% for >11 years. In this survey, vegans are usually young adults, mostly of a higher socioeconomic status and with an urban lifestyle. Interestingly, men and women were equally distributed. Various other studies have found predominantly moral, ethical, and ecological motivations, whereas health reasons are less frequently mentioned [2, 3].

A vegetarian diet is generally defined as a plant-based diet omitting meat and fish, whereas in a vegan diet no foods of animal origin, including milk, milk products, eggs, and honey are included. Definitions of subcategories of vegetarian and vegan diets in the scientific literature are summarized in Table 1.

In young children and adolescents, not only weight and height but also neurocognitive and psychomotor development are strongly influenced by the form and quality of their nutrition. Dietary influences on the intestinal microbiota may also influence epigenetic phenomena, allergic predisposition, and emotional and cognitive aspects of a person [4, 5]. Furthermore, the type of diet in infancy influences eating behavior later in life [6].

There is hardly any evidence that a vegan diet started early in childhood brings lasting health benefits [1, 7, 8]. Whereas studies on short-term outcome, such as coverage of macro- and micronutrients are relatively easily performed, studies on long-term health benefits are much more difficult to carry out. There are many confounders influencing long-term outcomes and incidence of chronic disease, vegans being in general more health-conscious, smoke less, are leaner, and physically more active [1]. Moreover, a vegan diet is a negative definition – it describes what is excluded from the diet – but what is actually eaten can be very heterogeneous, much depending on the options of the cultural and economical environment.

In a systematic review with meta-analysis of observational studies of adult cohorts, a plant-based diet was beneficial in terms of a reduction in chronic noncommunicable diseases such as obesity, type 2 diabetes, cardiovascular diseases, and some types of cancer [9]. The question remains whether this effect is due to the fact that animal products are avoided or whether this is to be attributed to a higher plant food intake. Another systematic review showed a dose-dependent risk reduction for coronary heart disease, stroke, total cancer, and all-cause mortality in correlation with daily fruit and vegetable consumption [10].

The only systematic review of studies on dietary intake and nutritional or health status of vegetarian and vegan infants, children, and adolescents was published in 2017 by Schürmann et al. [7]. They reviewed 24 publications from Western countries, among which there were only 2 studies of children on a vegan diet [11, 12]. The British collective of 39 children who were supplemented with vitamin B12 and vitamin D had on average a lower caloric intake (up to 300 kcal/day), whereas vitamin B12 and iron intakes exceeded the reference values [11]. In the larger US study with 404 young children who continued to receive supplementation after weaning, the children's physical development was within the reference range. The smaller height at 0–3 years of, on average, 2 cm, compared to the reference population, approached the 50th percentile at 10 years [12]. Neither study analyzed biomarkers. This systematic review by Schürmann et al. [7] revealed large study heterogeneity, generally small sample size often without control group, a trend toward upper social classes as a potential bias, and a peak of data stemming from the 1980s to the 1990s, which may limit the relevance of the findings to the present. The authors concluded that the existing data would not allow drawing any firm conclusions on the health benefits or risks of a vegetarian or vegan diet on the nutritional or health status of children in industrialized countries.

Nutrient Coverage of a Vegan Diet

In the following, we will briefly discuss the special nutritional aspects of a vegan diet. Plant-based nutrition is characterized by a rich coverage of β-carotene, vitamin C, folate, and magnesium as well as fiber and phytochemicals [13]. The latter are considered as protective modulators in the pathogenesis of inflammatory and carcinogenic processes [14]. On the other hand, a diet that completely dispenses with foods of animal origin is potentially critical in terms of energy, protein quality, long-chain fatty acids, iron, zinc, vitamin D, iodine, calcium, and especially vitamin B12 [1].

Awareness of these potentially critical nutrients allows parents who plan a vegan diet for themselves and their children to make informed decisions in their choice of foods and supplements.

Plant-based proteins have a less diversified amino acid composition than those from animals, so it is important to be aware of specific sources of different plant proteins and to increase intake in order to avoid a lack of essential amino acids. This is especially important as children require an approximately 30% higher intake for up to 2 years, 20–30% up to 6 years, and 15–20% for older children [15]. Vegan food sources generally have a higher fiber content and can thus lead to a deficit in the energy intake, particularly in infants and toddlers due to premature satiety and fullness. In this regard, attention needs to be paid to an adequate energy density of the food, good examples being pureed tofu or avocado, legumes, or cooked dried fruit. In the case of the vegan-fed infant, breast milk is generally recommended for at least the first 6 months of life, as with any newborn. If breastfeeding is not possible, a soy-based infant formula may be used. A systematic review published in 2014 concluded that soy-based infant formula is safe in terms of growth, metabolic, endocrinological, reproductive, and neurological functions [16]. However, compared to a cow's milk-based formula, soy-based milks have a higher concentration of phytates, aluminum, and phytoestrogens (isoflavones).

Essential polyunsaturated fatty acids such as omega-3 fatty acids, alpha-linolenic acid, eicosapentaenoic acid, and docosahexaenoic acid are vital for normal neurological development (e.g., synaptogenesis, retinal development). Since docosahexaenoic acid and eicosapentaenoic acid occur mainly in animal products, vegan children need to be sufficiently supplied with their alpha-linolenic acid precursor [17]. The inclusion of flaxseed, walnut, or rapeseed oil can prevent a shortage of omega-3 fatty acids.

In addition to its role in hemoglobin synthesis, iron is important for myelination of nerve sheaths and for neurotransmitter synthesis. Iron requirements in early childhood and adolescence are increased in comparison to adults. The bioavailability of heme iron (Fe^{2+}), which is typically found in meat, is better than that of nonheme iron (Fe^{3+}), the absorption of the latter being, depending on the food consumed at the same time, only between 2 and 20%. Therefore, care must be taken that inhibitors of iron absorption such as phytates from legumes, oxalic acids from rhubarb or spinach, and calcium compounds from milk are not taken simultaneously with important ferrous food sources. Conversely, it is known that ascorbic acid is a potent enhancer of nonheme iron absorption [18]. Zinc is also inhibited in its absorption by phytic acid. As an essential trace element and cofactor for many enzymes, clinical symptoms of zinc deficiency are diverse – in addition to impaired wound healing, nail brittleness, hair loss, or susceptibility to infection, possible consequences of a severe zinc deficiency are chronic diarrhea and impaired growth [19]. In the absence of food of animal origin, attention should be paid to sources of food rich in zinc such as cereals, fermented soy products, and nuts. For clinical zinc deficiency, additional supplementation is required (5 mg Zn/day for children 6–36 months, 10 mg Zn/day for older children) [20].

Although vitamin D is found in several foods of animal origin such as dairy products or fatty fish, the requirements of this vitamin are mainly covered by the endogenous production by UV-B irradiated skin. Use of fortified products or supplementation with 400–600 IU/day is recommended for all infants and toddlers [21]. The lack of milk and dairy products in the diet also reduces the supply of calcium, especially when the infant is weaned from breast milk or the (calcium-supplemented) soy-based infant formula. In the growing child, a sufficient calcium intake is important for the achievement of an optimal bone density (peak bone mass) and is a unique opportunity to reduce the risk of fractures and osteoporosis later in life. Green vegetables low in oxalate, such as broccoli, Chinese cabbage, collards, and kale, are good sources of calcium. Calcium-fortified drinks, cereals, and calcium-rich mineral water complete the food options [22].

As with other micronutrients, the content of iodine in breast milk depends on the nutritional status of the mother. In many countries, the use of iodine-supplemented salt is one of the most important factors to prevent previously endemic hypothyroidism. Particular attention should be paid to a sufficient supply of iodine to the baby, especially with self-prepared complementary foods [22].

Vitamin B12 (cobalamin) in a biologically active form is not available from non-animal sources and a vegan diet must therefore be regularly supplemented. Vitamin B12 is critical for the body to carry out many essential functions such as erythropoiesis, in myelin synthesis, axon homeostasis, and even mitochondrial energy metabolism. Deficiency, which may also occur in the breastfed child of a vitamin B12-deficient mother, may lead to severe, sometimes irreversible neuro-psychological damage and developmental delay [23, 24]. Laboratory assessment of vitamin B12 status plays a central role in the support of a vegan-fed child. Combining measurement of the vitamin substrate (holo-transcobalamin II having a higher sensitivity compared to cobalamin) together with measurement of methylmalonic acid in urine (as a sensitive metabolite of cobalamin metabolism) yields the best sensitivity and also excludes a functional cobalamin deficiency. The daily dose of cobalamin, which must be given orally as a supplement in infancy and childhood, is not yet established – suggestions recommend daily doses of 5 ug for infants and toddlers [25]. Some available commercial products use routes of administration such as nasal spray or toothpaste supplemented with vitamin B12 that are still under-studied for adequate absorption in childhood.

Recommendations and Conclusion

There are significant differences between the recommendations of the various nutrition and health associations worldwide, which in turn are probably due to the paucity and heterogeneity of available studies. North American nutrition and health organizations consider a well-balanced and well-planned vegan diet to be adequate to ensure healthy development at each stage of life including early childhood [26, 27]. However, European professional societies, such as the Swiss Federal Commission for Nutrition, the German Society for Nutrition and the European Society for Pediatric Gastroenterology, Hepatology and Nutrition, do not recommend a vegan diet during childhood [1, 28, 29]. If a vegan diet is chosen for ethical, ecological, or health reasons, a well-planned, diversified, adequate diet with additional supplementation of vitamin B12, vitamin D, iodine, and potentially other micronutrients is crucial to ensure a healthy and nutritious intake during childhood. The younger the child, the more we need to be critically aware of the potential dangers of a restrictive diet to the growing individual and, therefore, primarily advocate a diet that does not need to be supplemented [1]. At any age, a vegan diet requires profound nutritional knowledge from the parents and regular laboratory testing of the child. Qualified nutritional counseling and continuous pediatric medical support are indicated when a child is fed a vegan diet. Supporting tools, such as the recently developed food ex-

Table 2. Practical points to accompany children fed a vegan diet, adapted from [18]

In general
– Vegan diet accompanied by qualified dietician and pediatrician
– Explore motivation, discuss sources of information
– Collect a nutritional history, analyze a 3-day food diary, and regularly check critical nutrients (laboratory controls)
– Discuss supplements

Infants	Toddlers and children
Breastfed: if the mother is on a vegan/vegetarian diet, an nutritional evaluation is recommended (with analyses of critical micronutrients and potentially supplement them)	– Monitor energy intake (percentiles)
	– Limit raw food in toddlers (lower digestibility and caloric density)
Formula-fed: adapted soy-infant formula	– Check calcium intake (e.g., Ca-rich mineral water)
Complementary food	– Evaluate iodine supply (salt)
– BM or infant formula until 12 months	– Discuss vitamin B12 Supplement
– Pulses (puréed)/tofu is possible from 6 months onwards	– Check iron and vitamin D levels, possibly supplement
– Calorie dense solid food with oil supplemented (ALA-rich such as linseed, walnut, or rapeseed)	– Cave danger of aspiration (e.g., grinding nuts)
– Consider iron supplement (mainly in BM-fed infants after 6 months)	
– Vitamins K and D prophylaxis as all infants	
– Supplement vitamin B12 (after starting with complementary food)	

BM, breast milk; ALA, alpha-linolenic acid.

change systems for meal planning in vegan children, could be helpful in covering macro- and micronutritional needs [30]. A summary of aspects that need to be considered in the different age-groups is summarized in Table 2.

Disclosure Statement

The author has no conflicts of interest to declare.

References

1 Federal Commission for Nutrition (FCN). Vegan Diets: Review of nutritional benefits and risks. Expert report of the FCN. Bern: Federal Food Safety and Veterinary Office, 2018.

2 www.demoscope.ch/fileadmin/files/medienberichte/2017.03.15_Umfrage_Swissveg_Vegan_leben.pdf.

3 Janssen M, Busch C, Rödiger M, et al: Motives of consumers following a vegan diet and their attitudes towards animal agriculture. Appetite 2016; 105:643–651.

4 Paparo L, di Costanzo M, di Scala C, et al: The influence of early life nutrition on epigenetic regulatory mechanisms of the immune system. Nutrients 2014;6:4706–4719.

5 Prescott SL: Early nutrition as a major determinant of "immune health": Implications for allergy, obesity and other noncommunicable diseases. Nestle Nutr Inst Workshop Ser 2016;85:1–17.

6 Mennella JA, Ventura AK: Early feeding: setting the stage for healthy eating habits. Nestle Nutr Workshop Ser Pediatr Program 2011;68:153–163.

7 Schürmann S, Kersting M, Alexy U: Vegetarian diets in children: A systematic review. Eur J Nutr 2017;56:1797–1817.

8 Keller M, Müller S: Vegetarische und vegane ernährung bei kindern – stand der forschung und forschungsbedarf. Forsch Komplementmed 2016; 23:81–88.

9 Dinu M, Abbate R, Gensini GF, et al: Vegetarian, vegan diets and multiple health outcomes: a systematic review with meta-analysis of observational studies. Crit Rev Food Sci Nutr 2017;57: 3640–3649.

10 Aune D, Giovannucci E, Boffetta P, et al: Fruit and vegetable intake and the risk of cardiovascular disease, total cancer and all-cause mortality-a systematic review and dose-response meta-analysis of prospective studies. Int J Epidemiol 2017; 46:1029–1056.

11 Sanders TA: Growth and development of British vegan children. Am J Clin Nutr 1988;48:822–825.

12 O'Connell JM, Dibley MJ, Sierra J, et al: Growth of vegetarian children: The farm study. Pediatrics 1989;84:475–481.

13 Craig WJ: Health effects of vegan diets. Am J Clin Nutr 2009;89:1627S–1633S.

14 Fraga CG, Croft KD, Kennedy DO, et al: The effects of polyphenols and other bioactives on human health. Food Funct 2019;10:514–528.

15 Messina V, Mangels AR: Considerations in planning vegan diets: children. J Am Diet Assoc 2001; 101:661–669.

16 Vandenplas Y, Castrellon PG, Rivas R, et al: Safety of soya-based infant formulas in children. Br J Nutr 2014;111:1340–1360.

17 Craddock JC, Neale EP, Probst YC, Peoples GE: Algal supplementation of vegetarian eating patterns improves plasma and serum docosahexaenoic acid concentrations and omega-3 indices: a systematic literature review. J Hum Nutr Diet 2017;30:693–699.

18 Van Winckel M, Vande Velde S, De Bruyne R, Van Biervliet S: Clinical practice: vegetarian infant and child nutrition. Eur J Pediatr 2011;170: 1489–1494.

19 Roohani N, Hurrell R, Kelishadi R, Schulin R: Zinc and its importance for human health: An integrative review. J Res Med Sci 2013;18:144–157.

20 Brown KH, Rivera JA, Bhutta Z, et al: International Zinc Nutrition Consultative Group (IZiNCG) technical document #1. Assessment of the risk of zinc deficiency in populations and options for its control. Food Nutr Bull 2004;25(1 suppl 2):S99–S203.

21 EFSA Panel on Dietetic Products, Nutrition and Allergies (NDA): Dietary reference values for vitamin D. EFSA J 2016;14:4547.

22 Baroni L, Goggi S, Battaglino R, et al: Vegan nutrition for mothers and children: practical tools for healthcare providers. Nutrients 2018;11: pii E5.

23 Honzik T, Adamovicova M, Smolka V, et al: Clinical presentation and metabolic consequences in 40 breastfed infants with nutritional vitamin B12 deficiency – what have we learned? Eur J Paediatr Neurol 2010;14:488–495.

24 Dror DK, Allen LH: Effect of vitamin B12 deficiency on neurodevelopment in infants: current knowledge and possible mechanisms. Nutr Rev 2008;66:250–255.

25 Agnoli C, Baroni L, Bertini I, et al: Position paper on vegetarian diets from the working group of the Italian Society of Human Nutrition. Nutr Metab Cardiovasc Dis 2017;27:1037–1052.

26 Melina V, Craig W, Levin S: Position of the academy of nutrition and dietetics: vegetarian diets. J Acad Nutr Diet 2016;116:1970–1980.

27 Amit M: Canadian Paediatric Society: vegetarian diets in children and adolescents. Paediatr Child Health 2010;15:303–314.

28 Richter M, Boeing H, Grünewald-Funk D, et al; for the German Nutrition Society (DGE): Vegan diet. position of the German Nutrition Society (DGE). Ernährungs Umschau 2016;63:92–102.

29 Fewtrell M, Bronsky J, Campoy C, et al: Complementary feeding: a position paper by the European Society for Paediatric Gastroenterology, Hepatology, and Nutrition (ESPGHAN) committee on nutrition. J Pediatr Gastroenterol Nutr 2017;64:119–132.

30 Menal-Puey S, Martínez-Biarge M, Marques-Lopes I: Developing a Food Exchange System for Meal Planning in Vegan Children and Adolescents. Nutrients 2018;11:pii:E43.

Michaelsen KF, Neufeld LM, Prentice AM (eds): Global Landscape of Nutrition Challenges in
Infants and Children. Nestlé Nutr Inst Workshop Ser, vol 93, pp 111–120, (DOI: 10.1159/000503347)
Nestlé Nutrition Institute, Switzerland/S. Karger AG., Basel, © 2020

Role of Optimized Plant Protein Combinations as a Low-Cost Alternative to Dairy Ingredients in Foods for Prevention and Treatment of Moderate Acute Malnutrition and Severe Acute Malnutrition

Mark Manary · Meghan Callaghan-Gillespie

Department of Pediatrics, Washington University School of Medicine, St. Louis, MO, USA

Abstract

Tackling the global burden of acute malnutrition in children remains a major public health challenge and is essential for achieving sustainable development. Despite having effective treatment options, most wasted children go untreated; treatment coverage for severe acute malnutrition (SAM) children is only about 20%. Milk is currently an essential component of effective SAM treatment, incorporated into ready-to-use therapeutic food (RUTF). Reaching the untreated children, as well as preventing SAM, requires investment in innovative and cost-efficient approaches. To date, attempts to replace or remove milk from RUTF have been either unsuccessful or unpersuasive. This is likely because milk provides the highest protein quality and density of all typical RUTF ingredients. However, alternative protein sources could provide cost savings. Alternative protein sources, especially plant-based protein alternatives, have had shown more promising progress for the treatment of children with moderate acute malnutrition. Acknowledging that cost is a major barrier to the scale-up of treatment of acute malnutrition and that alternative protein sources are a practical means to reduce cost, continued research focusing on alternative proteins is necessary.

© 2020 Nestlé Nutrition Institute, Switzerland/S. Karger AG, Basel

Background

In 2017, prevalence surveys identified >50 million wasted children worldwide, defined as a weight-for-height Z-score less than –2 of World Health Organization's (WHO) Child Growth Standards [1]. Wasting leaves millions of children at an increased risk of illness and death, which continues to drive a global urgency for cost-effective solutions appropriate for scaling up treatment and prevention of wasting. Severe acute malnutrition (SAM), the most detrimental form of wasting, affects <17 million children under-5, and with an 11.6-fold increased risk for mortality than a non-wasted child, it was the cause of death for 3.5 million children worldwide [2]. Wasted children also experience an increased number of infectious diseases, delayed cognitive development, decreased adult stature, and reduced economic productivity [3, 4].

Cases of malnutrition are concentrated in sub-Saharan Africa and Asia, where chronic poverty is common [5]. In these regions, staple foods are often low in micronutrients and protein and families have limited access to health care and often consume inadequate diets [6]. The primary source of income for many of the families living in sub-Saharan Africa is subsistence farming, with the typical staple foods being starches like cassava, maize, and potatoes. Rice and wheat predominate as staples in south Asia.

SAM Treatment

The burden of SAM, while being inexcusably prevalent and often fatal, does have an effective; treatment, ready-to-use therapeutic food (RUTF), which is WHO. RUTF is a micronutrient-fortified, high-lipid (45–60% total energy), high-protein (10–12% total energy), energy-dense food (520–550 kcal/100 g) [7]. RUTF was created by replacing about half of the dried skimmed milk in the therapeutic milk formula with peanut paste, a food that provides generous amounts of fat and protein [8]. RUTF is a safe and highly effective treatment for children with acute malnutrition.

Despite its success and relative cost-effectiveness, <20% of children with SAM have access to treatment. One of the major barriers to scale-up of treatment is the high cost, of which more than a third comes from RUTF. One obstacle in the cost reduction of the standard RUTF (S-RUTF) formulation is the current UN agency specification that requires 50% of protein to come from dairy, the most expensive ingredient in RUTF. Recipients of RUTF are nutritionally vulnerable children with diets that lack food and consist of staple crops limited in the adequate dietary protein and essential amino acids (AAs) needed for vital human functions, including new tissue growth and vital organ recovery. To date, attempts to replace or remove milk have been either less successful or unpersuasive, but alternative protein sources continue to emerge as a clear productive path toward cost savings.

Moderate Acute Malnutrition Treatment

Children with moderate acute malnutrition (MAM) are defined as a weight-for-height Z-score less than or equal to –2, but greater than –3 and/or mid-upper arm circumference <12.5 to ≥11.5 cm [9]. These children, although suffering from a less severe wasting, also face an increased risk for death, susceptibility to infection, and long-term developmental consequences related to physical and intellectual productivity as adults. Evidence supports the notion that effective treatment of MAM prevents SAM, with data showing that in regions where MAM has been effectively treated, there are significant reductions in the severity and incidence of SAM [10].

The standard treatment for children with MAM is a food supplement made up of fortified blended flours. The most common is a corn-soya blend (CSB) that can often be made with from locally available, low-cost ingredients that are culturally and organoleptically acceptable in many settings. Because of concerns surrounding CSB, due to its low micronutrient content and bioavailability and antinutrient content, a modified dose of RUTF was recommended as a ready-to-use supplementary food (RUSF). The recovery rates using the classic CSB were < 75%, lower than those achieved with RUSF, which has prompted the World Food Programme and other food aid organizations to develop alternative MAM treatment foods. One CSB blend aimed to bridge the gap between RUSF and CSB is Super Cereal Plus that contains corn flour, soy flour, soy oil, dried skim milk, and concentrated minerals and vitamins. Similarly, alternative lower cost RUSF formulations that eliminate or reduce the dairy content have been developed and tested for the treatment of MAM. To date, there is still no consensus on the most effective treatment for MAM and the role of ingredient factors such as dairy.

Alternative SAM Treatments

In the last 2 decades, since the advent of home-based feeding and RUTF, there has been a growing demand for innovative and alternative treatment options to improve the coverage of treatment of acute malnutrition. Since skim milk powder is the most expensive ingredient in RUTF and its local availability in many of the countries where SAM is most prevalent is minimal, there have been focused efforts to substitute skim milk powder with alternative plant protein sources that are more readily available.

The most notable difference between plant protein and animal protein is the AA content. Protein is not a homogenous nutrient in which there is simply a dietary quantity needed, but rather protein is a collection of AAs. The role of the protein is determined by its distinctive combination of AAs; primarily the charge and configuration of the AAs. There are 21 different AAs that commonly comprise proteins [11]. There are 9 AAs that cannot be synthesized in the body, they are called essential AA, and need to be acquired through dietary sources [12], while the other AAs can be synthesized endogenously and considered nonessential.

Since the availability of AAs is equal to the sum of what the diet provides plus what can be synthesized, the distinction between essential and nonessential can be misleading. The AA requirement of wasted children is such that only 4 AAs can be met by endogenous synthesis. The body's protein is in a constant flux, degradation, and synthesis, requiring a steady supply of dietary AA to ensure all proteins can be assembled and execute their vital functions for optimal health [13]. For this reason, animal protein, such as milk, which contains considerable quantities of all AAs, has been recognized as the best protein source for wasted children. To date, most of the evidence validates this notion that animal protein, particularly milk protein, promotes the most growth and recovery in SAM children.

The 2010 study by Oakley et al. [14] was the first to consider using less milk in RUTF. This was a randomized, double-blind controlled clinical trial among 1,874 Malawian children with SAM who received either an isonitrogenous alternative RUTF containing 10% milk powder or S-RUTF (25% milk powder). Recovery was the primary outcome and was superior in the S-RUTF group when compared to the alternative RUTF, 84 and 81%, and survival analysis indicated that receiving 25% milk RUTF was associated with a higher rate of recovery ($p < 0.05$). Rates of weight gain were also significantly higher with S-RUTF ($p < 0.001$). Although the difference may seem modest to the public health community, it was caused by the increased milk content in S-RUTF.

A 2017 study challenged the supremacy of milk protein in RUTF. A clinical trial conducted in Malawi tested the efficacy of a milk-free, AA-enriched soya, sorghum, maize RUTF in a daily supervised setting and proved noninferiority to S-RUTF at a recovery level of 10% in SAM [15]. The recovery rate for both groups of children was 79%; however, the study population was atypical for SAM children in that 40% were over 2 years of age; typical 80–90% of SAM children are under 2 years of age and often under 1 year of age. Similar studies prior to this, conducted in Zambia and Democratic Republic of Congo, used the same milk-free RUTF formulation apart from the enrichment of the crystalline AAs

Table 1. Summary of all clinical treatment trials for SAM in children which utilize plant proteins as substitute for milk proteins

Study	Plant protein utilized	Milk protein, %	Population	Age (% <24 months)	Recovery, %	Weight Gain[†], g·kg⁻¹·day⁻¹, mean ± SD	Conclusions
Oakley et al. [14]	Soy	10	Malawi	83	81.0	1.94 ± 2.70	S-RUTF increased survival and weight gain compared to RUTF with 10% milk and soy
Irena et al. [16]	Soy, maize, sorghum	0	Zambia	82	53.3	2.2 ± 3.1	ITT analyses showed recovery and weight gain of the no-milk RUTF to be inferior to S-RUTF
Bahwere et al. [17]	Soy, maize, sorghum	0	Democratic Republic of Congo	47	72.9	Not available	In children >23 months, the no-milk RUTF was not inferior; however, in children 6–23 months, it was inferior
Bahwere et al. [17]	Soy, maize, sorghum + crystalline amino acids	0	Malawi	61	78.5	$6.5 \pm 4.2^{\ddagger}$	ITT analysis showed enriched amino acid, no-milk RUTF was no inferior to S-RUTF for the recovery of SAM. Although it was inferior by predefined margin for weight gain in children 24–59 months compared to S-RUTF
Bahwere et al. [17]	Soy, maize, sorghum	9.3	Malawi	61	78.6	$7.0 \pm 4.5^{\ddagger}$	ITT analysis showed RUTF with 9.3% milk was not inferior to S-RUTF for recovery of SAM

† Mean weight gain.
‡ For only the children discharged as cured.
SAM, severe acute malnutrition; RUTF, ready-to-use therapeutic food; S-RUTF, standard RUTF; ITT, intention-to-treat.

that were used in the Malawi study. The Zambia study used a design that replicated typical operational outpatient treatment for SAM with weekly follow-up visits and unsupervised feeding at home. Investigators stated that the results were inconclusive, but the recovery rate was higher among children receiving the S-RUTF compared to soy-maize-sorghum RUTF ($p = 0.034$) [16]. The Congo study protocol was similar to that used in Malawi, requiring daily clinic attendance for feeding, and found that soy-maize-sorghum RUTF among children older than 24 months was not an inferior when compared to S-RUTF [17]. The investigators of this study suggest that the reason for this difference between age-groups is unclear, but it is likely that children <24 months with SAM have greater requirements of certain AAs that were more bioavailable in S-RUTF [17]. These studies also highlight the importance of vigilant attention to the protein adequacy of RUTF as determined by the AA needs of the consumer. Table 1 summarizes the clinical treatment trials for SAM children that utilized less than the WHO-recommended amount of milk protein.

There have been no clinical trials comparing alternative RUTF containing egg or fish protein with S-RUTF, although nutritionists have suggested such options. It is uncertain whether these would be equivalent to S-RUTF, but unlikely any cost saving would be realized, as both egg and fish are more expensive than plant proteins. Soy protein isolate is often proposed as a plant-based alternative because a breastmilk substitute is made with such and has been used as the primary food for young infants in the developed world. The cost of soy protein isolate is, however, greater than milk protein; its availability quite limited and this has not been considered for RUTF.

Alternative MAM Treatments

MAM is best treated with a supplementary food that provides the nutrients likely to be insufficient in the habitual diet, namely, essential AAs, essential fatty acids, and micronutrients. Supplements usually provide micronutrients by adding crystalline vitamins and minerals, but the protein and fat are provided by the food ingredients. Because MAM children are not as clinically compromised as SAM children, it is thought the composition of supplementary food is less critical to the MAM child's well-being and a wide variety of supplementary foods are commonly used. This type of thinking is not consistent with the basic understanding that AAs are essential dietary building blocks, and when inadequate quantities are present in the diet, the physiological status of the child is compromised. It is important to recognize that AA deficiencies due to limited diet diversity are also augmented by malabsorption due to poor gut health or diversion of AAs to mount an inflammatory response [18–20].

We would suggest that provision of all essential AAs be given in quantity of the recommended dietary intake for all supplementary foods used in MAM. If all protein is derived from plant sources, as is often the case, this requires incorporating >1 plant protein source and utilizing a legume as a component. Table 2 compares the essential AA content of 250 kcal portion of 14 common plant staple foods. This table illustrates the reality that if a diet is based solely on cereal- or grain-based plant proteins, it is likely that the child's diet does not provide the recommended AA requirements.

When considering ready-to-use foods in children with MAM, plant protein foods have similar anthropometric outcomes when compared to standard peanut-milk RUSF. In Burkina Faso, there was a trial treating children with MAM with variations of blended flours and lipid-based RUSFs with varying amounts of milk, milk-soy combinations, or no milk [21]. The results revealed that there were no recovery differences between soy isolate RUSF

Table 2. Composition of the essential AAs in 14 common staple plant foods, g/250 kcal of food

Food	Lysine	Methionine	Tryptophan	Phenylalanine	Valine	Leucine	Isoleucine	Threonine	Histidine
Cereal/Grain									
Rice	0.16	0.1	0.05	0.24	0.27	0.37	0.19	0.16	0.1
Wheat	0.26	0.15	0.12	0.45	0.43	0.65	0.35	0.28	0.22
Maize	0.15	0.12	0.04	0.28	0.26	0.71	0.19	0.17	0.18
Sorghum	0.12	0.1	0.07	0.31	0.27	0.76	0.22	0.22	0.12
Legume									
Peanut	0.41	0.14	0.11	0.59	0.48	0.74	0.4	0.39	0.29
Chickpea	0.91	0.18	0.13	0.73	0.57	0.97	0.58	0.51	0.37
Common bean	1.21	0.27	0.21	0.96	0.93	1.41	0.78	0.74	0.49
Cowpea	1.18	0.25	0.22	1.02	0.83	1.34	0.71	0.67	0.54
Soy	1.31	0.27	0.29	1.03	0.98	1.61	0.96	0.86	0.53
Tuber/Root									
Cassava	0.29	0.07	0.08	0.22	0.25	0.3	0.21	0.2	0.12
Potatoes	0.32	0.08	0.08	0.23	0.3	0.32	0.22	0.19	0.12
Sweet potatoes	0.19	0.08	0.09	0.26	0.25	0.27	0.16	0.24	0.09
Yams	0.13	0.04	0.03	0.15	0.13	0.2	0.11	0.11	0.07
Skimmed milk	1.70	0.54	0.31	1.06	1.50	2.14	1.40	1.01	0.57

AAs, amino acids.

and milk protein RUSF ($p > 0.65$) [21]. The 20% milk RUSF did have a greater fat-free mass index compared to the 0% milk RUSF, although this was not statistically significant [21]. Similar recovery rates were seen in a Malawi study that treated children with MAM, with no significant differences in recovery among children receiving a soy/peanut RUSF and a soy protein isolate/whey RUSF, $p > 0.03$ [22]. Whereas a more recent trial in Malawi with a similar soy/peanut RUSF had lower recovery compared to a soy flour/whey RUSF in the treatment of MAM children, although both recovery rates were above 80% [23].

One area of recent concern, given the wide variety of supplementary food options, are the long-term consequences of supplemental feeding among children suffering from MAM. Recovered MAM children remain at a higher risk of relapsing and may require multiple periods of supplementary feeding and are more likely to suffer from nutritional deficits such as stunting [24]. A fear that distributing high-energy food supplements to treat MAM may promote unhealthy weight gain and increase risk of overweight or obesity has led to further investigation into the body composition effects of MAM treatment. However, limited evidence suggests that lipid-based nutrient supplement create *more lean body tissue* when compared to blended flour supplement, although further investigation into the role of milk compared to soy in lipid nutrient supplements is still needed [21]. This highlights the demand for supplements that provide a full range of nutrients for the synthesis of muscle and organ tissue and therefore prioritize fat-free tissue accretion.

Conclusion

Less expensive and more sustainable treatment options for the treatment of acute malnutrition are greatly desired but are yet to be realized. Milk-free SAM treatments have failed to prove their relevance as a noninferior alternative in an operational home-based treatment setting. It is essential to gain a better understanding of the suboptimal effectiveness of alternative formulations tested so far to help provide ways forward for optimization. Clinical trials with generalizable study populations and operational feeding protocols are essential for establishing pertinent noninferiority evidence. Crystalline AA supplementation may merit further exploration into the feasibility, cost, food safety, and stability.

Plant protein alternatives have a more prominent role in the treatment of children suffering from MAM. However, a more nuanced guideline that accounts for AA requirements during MAM is needed. This guideline would emphasize the necessity of combining different plant-based proteins to ensure the optimal quantities of AAs utilized. In addition to offering guidance to food-aid producers, these protein adequacy guidelines would also support appropriate and specific nutrition counseling for caregivers. Research to test the efficacy of treatment options in well-design clinical trials is necessary. Studies of the body composition effects of supplementary foods are also encouraged. Finally, the role of bioactives and other nonnutrient factors in animal source foods should not be neglected and further investigation into the short- and long-term advantages should be assessed and cost impact examined.

Disclosure Statement

The authors have no conflicts of interests to declare.

References

1 United Nations Children's Fund, WHO, The World Bank., Levels and Trends in Child Malnutrition. 2018. 2018 Edition.

2 Olofin I, McDonald CM, Ezzati M, et al: Associations of suboptimal growth with all-cause and cause-specific mortality in children under five years: a pooled analysis of ten prospective studies. PLoS One 2013;8:e64636.

3   Waber DP, Bryce CP, Girard JM, et al: Impaired
    IQ and academic skills in adults who experienced
    moderate to severe infantile malnutrition: a 40-
    year study. Nutr Neurosci 2014;17:58–64.
4   Black RE, Victora CG, Walker SP, et al: Maternal
    and child undernutrition and overweight in low-
    income and middle-income countries. Lancet
    2013;382:427–451.
5   Ijarotimi OS: Determinants of childhood malnu-
    trition and consequences in developing countries.
    Curr Nutr Rep 2013;2:129–133.
6   Pelletier B, Hickey G, Bothi KL, Mude A: Linking
    rural livelihood resilience and food security: An
    international challenge. Food Secur 2016;8:469–
    476.
7   Caron O: RUTF product specifications; in UNI-
    CEF SD, RUTF Pre-Bid Conference, MSF/Unicef,
    August, 2012.
8   Manary MJ, et al: Home based therapy for severe
    malnutrition with ready-to-use food. Arch Dis
    Child 2004;89:557–561.
9   Onis M: WHO Child growth standards based on
    length/height, weight and age. Acta Paediatrica
    2007;95:76–85.
10 Annan RA, Webb P, Brown R: Management of
    moderate acute malnutrition (MAM): current
    knowledge and practice; in CMAM Forum Tech-
    nical Brief, 2014.
11 Young VR: Protein and Amino Acids. In: Gersh-
    win ME, German JB, Keen CL (eds): Nutrition
    and Immunology. Humana Press, Totowa, NJ,
    Springer 2000, pp 49–64.
12 Joint FAO/WHO/UNU Expert Consultation on
    Protein and Amino Acid Requirements in Hu-
    man Nutrition, 2002, Geneva S, et al: Protein and
    Amino Acid Requirements in Human Nutrition:
    Report of a Joint FAO/WHO/UNU Expert Con-
    sultation, 2007.
13 Millward DJ: An adaptive metabolic demand
    model for protein and amino acid requirements.
    Br J Nutr 2003;90:249–260.
14 Oakley E, Reinking J, Sandige H, et al: A ready-
    to-use therapeutic food containing 10% milk is
    less effective than one with 25% milk in the treat-
    ment of severely malnourished children. J Nutr
    2010;140:2248–2252.
15 Bahwere P, Akomo P, Mwale M, et al: Soya,
    maize, and sorghum-based ready-to-use thera-
    peutic food with amino acid is as efficacious as
    the standard milk and peanut paste-based formu-
    lation for the treatment of severe acute malnutri-
    tion in children: a noninferiority individually
    randomized controlled efficacy clinical trial in
    Malawi. Am J Clin Nutr 2017;106:1100–1112.

16 Irena AH, Bahwere P, Owino VO, et al: Compari-
    son of the effectiveness of a milk-free soy-maize-
    sorghum-based ready-to-use therapeutic food to
    standard ready-to-use therapeutic food with 25%
    milk in nutrition management of severely acutely
    malnourished Zambian children: an equivalence
    non-blinded cluster randomised controlled trial.
    Matern Child Nutr 2015;11(suppl 4):105–119.
17 Bahwere P, Balaluka B, Wells JC, et al: Cereals
    and pulse-based ready-to-use therapeutic food as
    an alternative to the standard milk- and peanut
    paste-based formulation for treating severe acute
    malnutrition: a noninferiority, individually ran-
    domized controlled efficacy clinical trial. Am J
    Clin Nutr 2016;103:1145–1161.
18 Owino V, Ahmed T, Freemark M, et al: Environ-
    mental Enteric Dysfunction and Growth Failure/
    Stunting in Global Child Health. Pediatrics 2016;
    138:pii:e20160641.
19 Semba RD, Shardell M, Trehan I, et al: Metabolic
    alterations in children with environmental enter-
    ic dysfunction. Sci Rep 2016;6:28009.
20 Reeds PJ: Do the differences between the amino
    acid compositions of acute-phase and muscle
    proteins have a bearing on nitrogen loss in trau-
    matic states? J Nutr 1994;124:906–910.
21 Fabiansen C, Yaméogo CW, Iuel-Brockdorf AS, et
    al: Effectiveness of food supplements in increas-
    ing fat-free tissue accretion in children with mod-
    erate acute malnutrition: a randomised $2 \times 2 \times 3$
    factorial trial in Burkina Faso. PLoS Med 2017;
    14:e1002387.
22 LaGrone LN, Trehan I, Meuli GJ, et al: A novel
    fortified blended flour, corn-soy blend "plus-
    plus," is not inferior to lipid-based ready-to-use
    supplementary foods for the treatment of moder-
    ate acute malnutrition in Malawian children. Am
    J Clin Nutr 2012;95:212–219.
23 Stobaugh HC, Ryan KN, Kennedy JA, et al: In-
    cluding whey protein and whey permeate in
    ready-to-use supplementary food improves re-
    covery rates in children with moderate acute mal-
    nutrition: a randomized, double-blind clinical
    trial. Am J Clin Nutr 2016;103:926–933.
24 Stobaugh HC, Bollinger LB, Adams SE, et al: Ef-
    fect of a package of health and nutrition services
    on sustained recovery in children after moderate
    acute malnutrition and factors related to sustain-
    ing recovery: a cluster-randomized trial. Am J
    Clin Nutr 2017;106:657–666.

Michaelsen KF, Neufeld LM, Prentice AM (eds): Global Landscape of Nutrition Challenges in
Infants and Children. Nestlé Nutr Inst Workshop Ser, vol 93, pp 121–123, (DOI: 10.1159/000503565)
Nestlé Nutrition Institute, Switzerland/S. Karger AG., Basel, © 2020

Summary on the Role of Milk in Early Life

Human milk and cow's milk have crucial roles in early nutrition. According to WHO, breastfeeding is recommended to about the age of 2 years. However, when breastfeeding is terminated, cow's milk and dairy products are important to maintain optimal growth. The overall aim of this session was to cover different aspects of the effects of milk during early life, including the adverse effects if milk intake is very low and the use of cow's milk in foods given to children to prevent or treat undernutrition.

Lindsay Allen kicked this session off by giving an overview of human milk as the first source of micronutrients [1]. It is assumed that well-nourished mothers produce milk with adequate concentrations of micronutrients. However, some micronutrients are dependent on the diet of the mother and her use of supplements. Many of the recommended adequate intakes for intake of micronutrients for infants are based on poor data. Thus, it is difficult to assess the adequate intakes for infants. There is therefore a need for better reference data for micronutrients content in milk from well-nourished mothers. Such data should be based on studies including mothers from different areas of the world. *Lindsay Allen* gave a short introduction to the ongoing study (Mothers, Infants and Lactational Quality study) which she is in charge of. The study collects data from mother infant pairs in Bangladesh, The Gambia, Brazil, and Denmark with the main aim of establishing reference data for nutrients in human milk. She discussed the available knowledge of the concentration in human milk of several of the most important micronutrients. This included B12, which is dependent on the amount of cow's milk and animal foods in the diet of the mother and is important for cognitive development of the infant. The role of B12 in early life was also discussed in the presentations by *Yajnik Chittaranjan* and *Pascal Müller* in this session.

In the second presentation, *Kim F. Michaelsen* gave an overview on how cow's milk can stimulate growth [2]. The presentation focused on young children beyond the age of 12 months but included also data about the effects of intake of cow's milk on growth later in childhood and the potential influence on adult stature. There is convincing evidence that cow's milk and dairy protein can stimulate linear growth and weight gain, most likely due to stimulation of lean mass accretion. This is especially the case in low-income countries where intake of dairy products is often low. Because of the strong effect on growth, dairy products are an important ingredient in foods for preventing and treating undernutrition. UN organizations recommend that dairy protein should be included in foods for the treatment of severe acute malnutrition (SAM). However, due to the high cost of milk ingredients, foods with no or limited amounts of milk are considered for the treatment of moderate acute malnutrition (MAM). This was discussed in detail in the last presentation in this session by Mark Manary. A very high milk intake, especially during the second year of life, can have negative effects. It can increase the risk of later obesity because of the high protein intake and will reduce dietary diversity and increase the risk of iron deficiency.

Children not being breastfed and receiving no or only small amounts of cow's milk are at risk of B12 deficiency. In the third talk, *Yajnik Chittaranjan* talked about intergenerational aspects of vitamin B12 status [3]. The data he presented are based on a large cohort from Pune in India, where many have subclinical vitamin B12 deficiency, due to a vegetarian diet with low intake of milk. Based on data from this cohort, the life-course evolution of B12 deficiency has been described. In addition to the consumption of milk, genetics, transplacental and lactational transfer, and rapid growth have been shown to influence B12 status. A new and exciting area is the link between B12 status and the microbiome. Some bacteria can synthesize B12, and studies with some probiotics have shown a small increase in B12 status. Yajnik Chittaranjan and his research group have initiated a large intervention study with B12 supplementation to adolescents to examine the effects of a better B12 status for their future infants. Results from this intervention are not yet available.

Vitamin B12 deficiency was also a core issue in the fourth talk by *Pascal Müller* [4]. It was on vegan diet in young children. There is a rapid increasing trend in Europe with more and more families choosing to live on a vegan diet. If infants and young children are not receiving appropriate supplements with especially B12, but also with vitamin D, iodine, and other nutrients, they can develop severe deficiencies. Pascal Müller was co-author of a comprehensive Swiss expert report reviewing the nutritional benefits and risks of a vegan diet. While there might be benefits of a vegan diet in adults, several reports have concluded that there is hardly any evidence that a vegan diet early in childhood has beneficial health effects. His advice, in line with the ESPGHAN society, the German Society for Nutrition, and the Swiss report, was that a vegan diet should not be recommended for children. If parents insist, it is important to understand that there is a need for profound nutritional counseling and regular laboratory testing. In addition to B12, there is also a need to focus on the following nutritional aspects of the diet of infants and young children on a vegan diet: energy intake, protein quality, long-chain fatty acids, iron, zinc, vitamin D, iodine, and calcium.

Mark Manary finished the session with the presentation: Role of optimized plant protein combinations as a low-cost alternative to dairy ingredients in food for the prevention and treatment of MAM and SAM [5]. Cow's milk ingredients are included in most of the products used for the prevention and treatment of MAM and SAM due to the well-documented growth-stimulating effects. However, because of the high cost of skim milk powder, the most expensive ingredient in ready-to-use therapeutic foods, there has been an increasing interest in producing alternative products with locally available and low-cost ingredients. The challenge is to find combinations of plant-based proteins that have an amino acid pattern, which has an optimal growth-stimulating effect. Mark Manary gave an overview of the more recent attempts to find alternative protein sources that can match the growth-promoting effect of foods with milk protein. A recent approach has also been to add crystalline amino acids to optimize the amino acid pattern. It is estimated that at present only 20% of children with SAM receive treatment. Therefore, it is important to find cost-effective solutions.

Kim F. Michaelsen

References

1 Allen LH, Hampel D: Human Milk as the First Source of Micronutrients. In: Michaelsen KF, Neufeld LM, Prentice AM (eds): Global Landscape of Nutrition Challenges in Infants and Children. Nestlé Nutr Inst Workshop Ser. Basel, Karger, 2020, vol 93, pp 67–76.

2 Grenov B, Larnkjaer A, Mølgaard C, Michaelsen KF: Role of Milk and Dairy Products in Growth of the Child. In: Michaelsen KF, Neufeld LM, Prentice AM (eds): Global Landscape of Nutrition Challenges in Infants and Children. Nestlé Nutr Inst Workshop Ser. Basel, Karger, 2020, vol 93, pp 77–90.

3 Chittaranjan Y: Vitamin B12: An Intergenerational Story. In: Michaelsen KF, Neufeld LM, Prentice AM (eds): Global Landscape of Nutrition Challenges in Infants and Children. Nestle Nutr Inst Workshop Ser. Basel, Karger, 2020, vol 93, pp 91–102.

4 Müller P: Vegan Diet in Young Children. In: Michaelsen KF, Neufeld LM, Prentice AM (eds): Global Landscape of Nutrition Challenges in Infants and Children. Nestlé Nutr Inst Workshop Ser. Basel, Karger, 2020, vol 93, pp 103–110.

5 Manary M, Callaghan-Gillespie M: Role of Optimized Plant Protein Combinations as a Low-Cost Alternative to Dairy Ingredients in Foods for Prevention and Treatment of MAM and SAM. In: Michaelsen KF, Neufeld LM, Prentice AM (eds): Global Landscape of Nutrition Challenges in Infants and Children. Nestlé Nutr Inst Workshop Ser. Basel, Karger, 2020, vol 93, pp 111–120.

Michaelsen KF, Neufeld LM, Prentice AM (eds): Global Landscape of Nutrition Challenges in
Infants and Children. Nestlé Nutr Inst Workshop Ser, vol 93, pp 125–131, (DOI: 10.1159/000503349)
Nestlé Nutrition Institute, Switzerland/S. Karger AG., Basel, © 2020

Environmental and Physiological Barriers to Child Growth and Development

Andrew M. Prentice

MRC Unit The Gambia at London School of Tropical Medicine and Hygiene, Banjul, The Gambia

Abstract

Aggregated analyses of child growth in low- and middle-income countries (LMICs) reveal a remarkably consistent picture of serious growth failure compared to the WHO reference growth curves. Impoverished diets with low dietary diversity are a key driver of poor growth, but there are important additional environmental factors that limit the uptake and utilization of nutrients. This paper considers such factors. A large proportion of the rapid growth deterioration in later infancy can be ascribed to infections and to wider nonspecific effects of living in an unhygienic environment, including the ingestion of toxins such as aflatoxin. Despite never revealing themselves as clinical syndromes, the great majority of children in rural low-income settings of Africa and Asia are antibody positive to numerous pathogens (CMV, EB, HepB, *Helicobacter pylori*, and many more) by 24 m; these infections must take their toll. Additionally, there is a syndrome widely termed environmental enteric disease that combines gut leakage with a chronic inflammation leading to nutrient losses and cytokine-mediated growth retardation. Systemic inflammation also inhibits nutrient uptake and utilization. Elimination of these environmental barriers will be key to achieving optimal child growth and development in LMICs.

Introduction

Multicountry analysis of child growth in low-income countries reveals a remarkably consistent picture of serious growth failure compared to the WHO reference growth curves [1]. Birth weight is generally lower by 0.5–1.0 Z-score. Young infants then grow reasonably well until about 3 m postpartum when they enter a period of precipitate decline compared to the WHO reference, such that population averages often reach –2 Z-scores and worse in the second year of life. By 24 m, this decline halts, and in many settings, there follows a period of gradual catch-up. Data from rural Gambia shown in Figure 1 reflect these trends and extend the analysis into adulthood [2].

The low birth weight often seen in poor populations, especially in Asia, can be ascribed in part to small maternal size that reflects the environmental effects in prior generations. Possible epigenetic mechanisms that might mediate these intergenerational effects are discussed by Silver elsewhere in this symposium [3].

After birth, young, fully breastfed infants tend to thrive for the first few months and often reclaim some of the deficit with which they were born. The subsequent growth faltering is caused in part by poor diets with low dietary diversity and by the consequent deficiencies in a wide range of nutrients, but this is not the only factor. The aim of this chapter is to highlight some of the additional environmental factors that create barriers to healthy child growth and development by impairing the utilization of nutrients. The effects of clinical infections are well known and have been extensively summarized elsewhere so are not reprised here [4]. Instead, we cover one well-known factor, namely, the effects of chronic environmental enteric disease (EED), and 3 lesser-known factors. The first of these relates to the more insidious effects of children's exposures to a wide range of pathogens that rarely, or never, manifest as clinical syndromes. The second is a summary of evidence about the effects of aflatoxin exposure on child growth. The third topic considers the effects of persistent low-grade systemic inflammation on nutrient uptake and utilization. The effects of dysbiosis of the gut microbiome are covered elsewhere in this volume [5].

The Possible Effects of "Silent" Subclinical Infections

A proportion of the rapid growth deterioration seen in later infancy and in the second year of life in low- and middle-income countries (LMICs) settings can be ascribed to overt infections such as diarrhea, malaria, and pneumonia. Par-

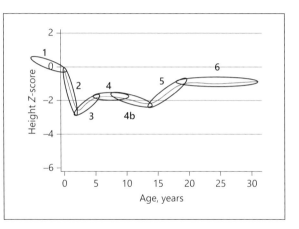

Fig. 1. Life course of stunting in rural Gambians. (1) Fetal growth retardation. (2) Precipitate decline from 3 to 24 months. (3) Spontaneous catch-up in preschoolers. (4) Stability in childhood. (4a) Artifactual decline as reference standard children enter puberty earlier. (5) Pubertal catch-up. (6) Adult status.

ents recognize the effects of such illnesses and seek medical care if available. Mothers in particular note the effects of such illnesses on their child's appetite. But there is a second category of infections whose possible impact on appetite and nutrient utilization is rarely considered. These "silent" subclinical infections rarely reveal themselves as clinical syndromes. Yet, the majority of children in rural African settings are antibody positive to numerous pathogens (CMV, EB, HepB, *Helicobacter pylori*, and many more) by their first birthday. For instance, the prevalence of *H. pylori* infection in a study we conducted in rural Gambian infants was 56% at 12 months, but incidence rates were higher with some infants clearing their infection and then becoming reinfected [6]. CMV infection rates are notoriously high in young LMIC children, and this can be exacerbated by exposure to HIV [7]. The metabolic sequelae of these silent infections are unknown, but they must surely take their toll on metabolism and may have additional effects on the hormonal pathways regulating growth.

Environmental Enteric Disease

Additional to these silent infections and possibly related in part is a silent syndrome widely termed EED (Fig. 2) [8–11]. EED is a complex, common, and usually persistent damage to the gut mucosa. It combines villous atrophy with crypt hyperplasia, loss of tight junctions, and a chronic, nonresolving inflammatory infiltrate to the gut lining.

The etiology of EED is still not entirely clear and probably results from a constellation of factors all related to poverty and pooled under the label of water, sanitation, and hygiene (WASH). Pathogens causing diarrhea play a contribu-

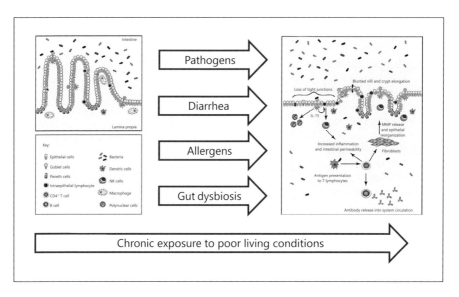

Fig. 2. Genesis and pathophysiology of environmental enteric disease (EED).

tory (though not necessarily dominant) role [8]. As described by Robertson in this session [5], alterations in the gut microbiota reflecting an inappropriately slow maturation toward the normal postinfancy profile [12] and/or a frank dysbiosis [5, 13] each may play an additional role.

The features of EED combine to cause nutrient malabsorption, nutrient leakage and losses, metabolic wastage in fuelling the chronic inflammation, and translocation of whole bacteria or their inflammatory debris. It is likely that these all conspire to drive cytokine-mediated growth retardation [7].

Aflatoxin Exposure

Aflatoxins represent a range of carcinogenic toxins produced primarily by Aspergillus fungi that grow on poorly stored grains and seeds especially in hot and humid tropical climes. Early-life aflatoxin exposure is an important risk factor for cancers, especially liver cancer in later life. Aflatoxin can also be immunosuppressive at high doses and there has been much interest in its possible impact on child growth, an impact that has been frequently demonstrated in animal studies.

Human observational studies have frequently shown an association between aflatoxin exposure and poor growth [14, 15] including in longitudinal analyses where, for instance, high maternal blood levels of aflatoxin adduct (a measure of persistent exposure) have been associated with slower growth in the offspring [16]. The plausibility of such a link has been reinforced by a recent study showing that epigenetic methylation patterns of certain genes in the growth axis (including insulin-like growth factor 1) measured in infants are correlated with aflatoxin levels in their mothers' blood during pregnancy [17]. However, all of these associations might be caused by confounding whereby poorer families have both higher exposure to aflatoxin and poorer growth in their children. It is also noteworthy that not all association studies show a linkage and one even shows a reverse association, thus emphasizing that we do not clearly understand whether aflatoxin does have direct effects on child growth. Randomized controlled intervention trials of aflatoxin reduction will be needed to clarify this picture, and, notably, a recent trial has reported a null effect on growth despite success in reducing aflatoxin exposure [18].

Notwithstanding a lack of definitive proof linking aflatoxin exposure to child growth, there is every reason to support efforts targeted at aflatoxin reduction and strategies such as biocontrol of the Aspergillus fungus show great promise.

Chronic Low-Grade Systemic Inflammation

Micronutrient deficiencies, which can impact on growth, and especially iron deficiency leading to anemia, can also be caused in some part by infections that impair both absorption and utilization of nutrients. Recent evidence suggests that a role for low-grade inflammation may be especially critical. The stress of birth is associated with a sharp and sort-lived increase in inflammation and then young infants generally display few signs of any inflammation. However, indicators of inflammation such as C-reactive protein and alpha-1 glycoprotein rise progressively in infancy in most LMIC populations. In rural Gambia, we have reported that, in different studies, 20–45% of infants over 2 months have C-reactive protein levels >5 mg/L and up to 80% have alpha-1 glycoprotein levels showing recent infection [6, 19].

The mechanism by which inflammation can cause a micronutrient deficiency has been most clearly demonstrated for iron where, in the presence of an infectious threat and/or the related inflammation, the iron-regulatory hormone hepcidin is upregulated by IL6 [20]. This blocks iron absorption in the duodenum and reduces circulating iron by locking it away in reticuloendothelial macrophages [20]. Recent evidence shows that many children living in a poor environment have persistently raised levels of hepcidin and that these elevated levels are driven by even very low-grade inflammation [21]. The source of this inflammation is still unclear, but it is apparent that respiratory infections are one important cause, leading to the novel and unexpected insight that inflammation in airways epithelia might be an important driver of iron deficiency and its consequent anemia.

Thresholds of Environmental Hygiene That Must Be Attained to Normalize Child Growth

An obvious conclusion arising from the above description of the diverse nutrition-sensitive contributors to poor child growth and development is that optimal growth will only be achieved within an optimal environment. Elsewhere in this volume, Humphrey summarizes the very disappointing results of recent WASH interventions that have endeavored to create such an environment [22]. Our own analysis of child growth in families across a very broad gradient of socioeconomic status and housing conditions suggests that there is a very high threshold of hygiene that must be reached before children will be free from the environmental inhibitors of adequate growth described in this paper [23]. This reinforces Humphrey's call for the so-called "Transformative WASH" solutions.

Future Prospects

The rapid decline in stunting and anemia rates seen in many South American countries in the past 3 or 4 decades has been well documented, especially in Brazil, where it seems clear that concerted efforts involving improved water and sanitation facilities, improvements in breast-feeding rates, poverty reduction, and mothers' education have all contributed to the excellent progress seen. Thus, we can be optimistic that the global metrics on childhood malnutrition will drastically improve as countries pass through the economic transition (albeit with a risk of overweight and obesity). The evidence presented here emphasizes the need for holistic approaches that encompass a wide range of environmental improvements in addition to nutrition-specific interventions.

Disclosure Statement

The author received travel support and an honorarium from the Nestlé Nutrition Institute (NNI) for this meeting. The author is a Board Member for (NNI).

References

1 Victora CG, de Onis M, Hallal PC, et al: World-wide timing of growth faltering: Revisiting implications for interventions. Pediatrics 2010; 125:e473–e480.

2 Prentice AM, Ward KA, Goldberg GR, et al: Critical windows for nutritional interventions against stunting. Am J Clin Nutr 2013;97:911–918.

3 Silver MJ: Intergenerational influences on child development: An epigenetic perspective. In: Michaelsen KF, Neufeld LM, Prentice AM (eds): Global Landscape of Nutrition Challenges in Infants and Children. Nestlé Nutr Inst Workshop Ser, vol 93, pp 145–151.

4 Guerrant RL, Schorling JB, McAuliffe JF, et al: Diarrhea as a cause and an effect of malnutrition: Diarrhea prevents catch-up growth and malnutrition increases diarrhea frequency and duration. Am J Trop Med Hyg 1992;47:28–35.

5 Robertson R: The gut microbiome in child malnutrition. In: Michaelsen KF, Neufeld LM, Prentice AM (eds): Global Landscape of Nutrition Challenges in Infants and Children. Nestlé Nutr Inst Workshop Ser, vol 93, pp 133–143.

6 Darboe MK, Thurnham DI, Morgan G, et al: Effectiveness of an early supplementation scheme of high-dose vitamin A versus standard WHO protocol in Gambian mothers and infants: a randomised controlled trial. Lancet 2007;369:2088–2096.

7 Evans C, Chasekwa B, Rukobo S, et al: Cytomegalovirus acquisition and inflammation in human immunodeficiency virus-exposed uninfected Zimbabwean infants. J Infect Dis 2017;215:698–702.

8 Harper KM, Mutasa M, Prendergast AJ, et al: Environmental enteric dysfunction pathways and child stunting: a systematic review. PLoS Negl Trop Dis 2018;12:e0006205.

9 Guerrant RL, DeBoer MD, Moore SR, et al: The impoverished gut – a triple burden of diarrhoea, stunting and chronic disease. Nat Rev Gastroenterol Hepatol 2013;10:220–229.

10 MAL-ED Network Investigators: Relationship between growth and illness, enteropathogens and dietary intakes in the first 2 years of life: findings from the MAL-ED birth cohort study. BMJ Glob Health 2017;2:e000370.

11 Owino V, Ahmed T, Freemark M, et al: Environmental enteric dysfunction and growth failure/stunting in global child health. Pediatrics 2016; 138 pii:e20160641.

12 Subramanian S, Huq S, Yatsunenko T, et al: Persistent gut microbiota immaturity in malnourished Bangladeshi children. Nature 2014;510: 417–421

13 Smith MI, Yatsunenko T, Manary MJ, et al: Gut microbiomes of Malawian twin pairs discordant for kwashiorkor. Science 2013;339:548–554.

14 Watson S, Moore SE, Darboe MK, et al: Impaired growth in rural Gambian infants exposed to aflatoxin: a prospective cohort study. BMC Public Health 2018;18:1247.

15 Lombard MJ: Mycotoxin exposure and infant and young child growth in Africa: What do we know? Ann Nutr Metab 2014;64(suppl 2):42–52.

16 Turner PC, Collinson AC, Cheung YB, et al: Aflatoxin exposure in utero causes growth faltering in Gambian infants. Int J Epidemiol 2007;36:1119–1125.

17 Hernandez-Vargas H, Castelino J, Silver MJ, et al: Exposure to aflatoxin B1 in utero is associated with DNA methylation in white blood cells of infants in The Gambia. Int J Epidemiol 2015;44: 1238–1248.

18 Hoffmann V, Jones K, Leroy JL: The impact of reducing dietary aflatoxin exposure on child linear growth: a cluster randomised controlled trial in Kenya. BMJ Glob Health 2018;3:e000983.

19 Armitage AE, Agbla SC, Betts M, et al: Rapid growth is a dominant predictor of hepcidin suppression and declining ferritin in Gambian infants. Haematologica 2019;104:1542–1553.

20 Ganz T: Systemic iron homeostasis. Physiol Rev 2013;93:1721–1741.

21 Prentice AM, Bah A, Jallow MW, et al: Respiratory infections drive hepcidin-mediated blockade of iron absorption leading to iron deficiency anemia in African children. Sci Adv 2019;5:eaav9020.

22 Makasi R, Humphrey JH: Summarizing the child growth and diarrhoea findings of the WASH Benefits and SHINE trials. In: Michaelsen KF, Neufeld LM, Prentice AM (eds): Global Landscape of Nutrition Challenges in Infants and Children. Nestlé Nutr Inst Workshop Ser, vol 93, pp 153–166.

23 Husseini M, Darboe MK, Moore SE, et al: Thresholds of socio-economic and environmental conditions necessary to escape from childhood malnutrition: a natural experiment in rural Gambia. BMC Med 2018;16:199.

Michaelsen KF, Neufeld LM, Prentice AM (eds): Global Landscape of Nutrition Challenges in
Infants and Children. Nestlé Nutr Inst Workshop Ser, vol 93, pp 133–143, (DOI: 10.1159/000503352)
Nestlé Nutrition Institute, Switzerland/S. Karger AG., Basel, © 2020

The Gut Microbiome in Child Malnutrition

Ruairi C. Robertson

Centre for Genomics and Child Health, Blizard Institute, Queen Mary University of London, London, UK

Abstract

Undernutrition affects almost 25% of all children under the age of 5 worldwide and underlies almost half of all child deaths. Child undernutrition is also associated with long-term
growth deficits, in addition to reduced cognitive potential, reduced economic potential,
and elevated chronic disease risk in later life. Dietary interventions alone are insufficient to
comprehensively reduce the burden of child undernutrition and fail to address the persistent infectious burden of the disease. Although the role of infections is well recognized in
the pathogenesis of undernutrition, an emerging body of evidence suggests that commensal microbial communities, known as the microbiome, also play an important role. The gut
microbiome regulates energy harvesting from nutrients, growth hormone signaling, colonization resistance, and immune tolerance against pathogens, amongst other pathways
critically associated with healthy child growth. Hence, disturbance of the normal gut microbial ecosystem via undernourished diets or unhygienic environments, especially in the early phases of life, may perturb these critical pathways associated with child growth, thereby
contributing to child undernutrition. Here we discuss the emerging evidence for the role of
the gut microbiome in child undernutrition and the potential for novel gut microbiota-
targeted treatments to restore healthy child growth.

The Global Burden of Child Malnutrition

Child undernutrition can be broadly classified as either stunting (length-for-age Z-score [LAZ] ≤2) or wasting (weight-for-height Z-score ≤2). However, other anthropometric and clinical measures including low head circumference, weight-for-age Z-score, or the presence of edema can also be used as indicators of undernutrition. Despite trends in child undernutrition declining substantially in the past 30 years, >50 million children are wasted and >150 million children (representing 22% of the entire global population under 5 years of age) are stunted [1]. Furthermore, absolute numbers affected by stunting are expected to rise in sub-Saharan Africa with population growth. It is estimated that undernutrition underlies 45% of all child deaths globally. Furthermore, child undernutrition is associated with long-term growth deficits, reduced cognitive potential, reduced economic potential, and elevated chronic disease risk in later life [2]. Hence, the burden of child undernutrition remains a significant threat to global public health.

The central dogma of undernutrition suggests that the disorder is solely treated and prevented through nutrition. However, recent estimates suggest that the 10 most effective nutrition interventions, if scaled up to 90% in high-burden countries, would only reduce stunting by 20% and wasting by 60% [3]. Hence, child undernutrition is increasingly viewed as a complex disorder driven by a number of nutritional, infectious, physiological, economical, and psychosocial factors. Each of these facets of undernutrition needs to be addressed in order to effectively reduce the mortality and morbidity associated with the disease.

Child Malnutrition as a Microbial Disorder

Stunting and wasting are clinically distinct as chronic and acute disease states, respectively; however, both forms of undernutrition share a number of metabolic phenotypes and pathogeneses. Both forms of undernutrition exhibit environmental enteric dysfunction (EED), a state of intestinal pathology characterized by blunted villi, inflammation, and reduced barrier function, among other enteropathic phenotypes [4]. EED is associated with reduced nutrient absorption and hence faltering growth phenotypes. The direct cause of EED is unknown; however, it is hypothesized that infection and subclinical pathogen carriage contribute to EED and undernutrition. Large, global, multicenter trials have reported that subclinical enteropathogen carriage is almost ubiquitous among children in low- to middle-income settings and that the number of carried enteropathogens is inversely associated with both weight and height [5–7]. Furthermore, infection is a common cause of death in outpatients following severe acute malnutrition (SAM) and is also strongly associated with faltered growth following SAM [8]. Antibiotics reduce mortality in regions of high undernutrition prevalence even in the absence of confirmed infections [9] and may also reduce stunting [10] and improve growth outcomes following SAM [11–13], although this evidence is conflicting.

These data provide strong evidence for a role of pathogenic microorganisms in both stunting and wasting. However, emerging data also provide evidence for the role of commensal gut microorganisms (gut microbiome) in metabolic disease states and in normal intestinal structure and function [14]. The gut microbiome plays a critical role in the integrity of the intestinal barrier, nutrient absorption, metabolic homeostasis, and immune maturity, particularly in the early stages of life. Disruption of the intestinal microbial environment via antibiotics, suboptimal nutrition, or unhygienic environments has been causally related to chronic intestinal and metabolic disease states. Due to known intestinal, metabolic, and immune pathologies in faltered child growth, these emerging data lend to the hypothesis of a role of the commensal microbiome in child undernutrition.

Succession of a Healthy Infant Gut Microbiome

The timing of infant microbiome acquisition remains under scientific debate. The sterile womb hypothesis has recently been challenged by conflicting reports of complex microbial communities in the placenta [15]. Comprehensive studies in experimental animals and humans have both refuted and supported the claim of a placental microbiome, and hence exposure to a prenatal microbiome, in recent years [16, 17]. Regardless of the timing of initial exposure, early postnatal events comprehensively determine the structuring of the infant microbiome in the early stages of life. Birth mode, early feeding practices, and antibiotic usage critically shape infant gut microbiome composition and function in the first 2–3 years of life [14]. Facultative anaerobes are typically the first colonizers of the infant gut followed by obligate anaerobes such as *Bifidobacteria* (particularly *B. longum*), *Bacteroides,* and *Clostridium,* which contain enzymes essential for the digestion of human milk oligosaccharides (HMO). In breastfed infants, *Bifidobacteria* compose a large proportion of the early infant microbiome. Weaning triggers an expansion of gut microbiome diversity, whereby *Faecalibacterium prausnitzii, Ruminococcus*, and other species involved in complex polysaccharide metabolism expand in relative abundance. By 2–3 years of age, the gut microbiome stabilizes to closely resemble that of an adult. This programmed maturation of the infant microbiome assembly, which is driven primarily by early-life feeding practices, is strongly predictive of healthy child growth [18].

The Microbiome of Stunting

The pathogenesis of stunting occurs within the first 1,000 days (the time period from conception to 2 years of age). Up to 20% of stunting is estimated to occur in utero, after which LAZ tend to remain stable during the first 6 months of life. From 6 months until 2 years of age, child LAZ tends to decline in regions of high stunting prevalence, coinciding with the cessation of breastfeeding and the introduction of solid foods [19]. The introduction of solid foods and exposure to other environmental microbes simultaneously triggers the rapid expansion of gut microbiome diversity during this period from 6 months to 2 years of age. Interestingly, the gut microbiota drives a weaning reaction that is critical for immune maturity and tolerance in later life, which play plausibly be related to growth and it's association with infectious burden [20]. It is hence hypothesized that gut microbiome maturation partially regulates linear growth during this time period and that dysregulation of gut microbiome structuring may contribute to early childhood stunting [14].

Child stunting has recently been associated with "decompartmentalization" of the intestinal tract, whereby microorganisms of oropharyngeal origin were more abundant in fecal samples of stunted children from sub-Saharan Africa [21]. The authors hypothesize that the overabundance of these organisms, including *Lactobacillus salivarius* and *Prevotella histicola* among others, trigger chronic inflammatory responses when present lower in the intestinal tract, outside of their ecological niche, thereby contributing to faltered linear growth. Although intestinal inflammation is a hallmark of stunting, it is not yet clear if it is driving EED and faltered growth or purely present as a consequence of intestinal and metabolic disturbance. Smaller studies in Malawi, Bangladesh, and India have also reported that stunting is associated with reduced *Bifidobacterium longum*, *Lactobacillus mucosae*, and alpha diversity as well as elevated *Acidaminococcus spp* abundance and glutamate fermentation pathways [22, 23].

A number of preclinical studies have shed light on the cause and effect of the gut microbiome and child stunting. A cocktail of Bacteroidales species and *Escherichia coli* in combination with an undernourished diet is capable of recapitulating the phenotypes of EED, reduced linear growth, and reduced pathogen tolerance in mice [24]. Conversely, specific strains of *Lactobacillus plantarum* can restore the linear growth deficits observed in germ-free mice via regulation of growth hormone and insulin-like growth factor 1, suggesting that the gut microbiome critically regulates endocrine pathways associated with early-life growth [25].

A causal role for the interaction between breast milk, enteropathogens, and the infant microbiome in stunted growth has also been demonstrated in mice.

Mothers of stunted infants produce fewer HMOs than mothers of healthy growing infants. HMOs are critically metabolized by the infant microbiome and are a major source of energy for infants. When a defined consortia of bacteria from a stunted infant's fecal sample was transplanted into germ-free animals, the mice displayed impaired growth that was recovered following supplementation with bovine milk oligosaccharides that were structurally similar to HMOs [26]. Milk oligosaccharides had no growth-promoting effect in germ-free mice, suggesting a microbiota-dependent effect on growth. Similarly, the growth-inhibiting effect of certain pathobionts may also be dependent on the larger gut microbiome community, whereby the pathobiont alone does not inhibit growth in experimental animals, but relies on the presence of a "stunted" microbiome [27].

The Microbiome of Wasting

Wasting is often considered a more acute state of undernutrition than stunting. However, the EED pathology of both wasting and stunting is similar. Severe wasting or SAM is defined as a WHZ greater than −3, mid upper-arm circumference <115 mm, or the presence of bilateral pitting edema. In complicated cases, SAM is treated in hospital settings and incurs high relapse and mortality despite standardized antibiotic and therapeutic feeding protocols [28]. It is hypothesized that the intestinal dysfunction observed in SAM contributes to nutrient malabsorption and immune dysfunction, which may be partially driven by a disturbed microbiome [14].

A metric of microbiome maturity, termed the microbiota-for-age Z-score, has been derived from a cohort of healthy growing infants in Bangladesh and validated in humans and experimental animals [17]. Disturbance of this programmed assembly of the gut microbiome in early life contributes to a state of microbiome "immaturity." It has been shown that reduced microbiome maturity or microbiota-for-age Z-score is strongly predictive of wasting in infants. Furthermore, therapeutic feeding following SAM only temporarily restores microbiome maturity, suggesting that the relapse of the microbiome to an immature state may predispose an infant to SAM relapse. Further statistical metrics have since been developed that identified microbiome 'ecogroups' consisting of 15 bacterial taxa, that exhibit consistent variation during the first 5 years of life that can robustly explain child growth [29]. Other cohorts have demonstrated a depletion of obligate anaerobes and the methanogenic archaeal species *Methanobrevibacter smithii* in SAM [30].

Preclinical models have further demonstrated the causality of a disturbed microbiome in SAM. A large twin cohort from Malawi identified no clear taxa differentiating healthy children from their undernourished twins; however, transplantation of stool from these children into germ-free mice transferred growth phenotypes [31]. These growth deficits appear to be restored through colonization of "undernourished" animals with a small consortium of microbes from the healthy twin [32]. Furthermore, the immunoglobulin A (IgA)-targeted fraction of the microbiome in SAM may be critical in growth faltering [33]. IgA appear to target Enterobacteriaceae in children with SAM, which leads to growth faltering and death when transplanted into germ-free mice. Conversely, the IgA-targeted fraction of the healthy infant microbiome appears to be dominated by *Akkermansia muciniphila*, a commensal involved in intestinal mucus maintenance, suggesting a distinct interaction between the infant microbiome, the maturing immune system, and growth.

Dietary Insufficiencies, Gut Microbiome, and Undernutrition

Macronutrient and micronutrient deficiencies undoubtedly contribute to faltered growth in infants; however, emerging evidence suggests that the gut microbiome may mediate the effect of diet on nutritional status through a number of mechanisms. Emerging evidence of these microbiome–nutrient interactions may help in the development of "microbiota-directed foods" to specifically target the impaired microbiome in child undernutrition.

Bacterial growth relies on specific metabolism of micronutrients, which in turn may influence host-microbe interactions relating to immune sensitivity and growth. Host vitamin A receptors have been well studied in the context of child undernutrition; however, less is known about the gut microbial interaction with dietary vitamin A. Recently, it was reported that dietary vitamin A deficiency appears to exert the most profound change on gut microbiota structure in experimental animals compared with zinc, iron, or folate deficiency [34]. Notably, it has been shown that the specific interaction between vitamin A metabolism and the growth-promoting bacterial taxon *Bacteroides vulgatus* may influence infant microbiota composition in the context of undernutrition. Due to the emerging evidence for the epigenetic influence in child undernutrition, the role of dietary methyl donors may be of importance. The dietary deficiency of methyl donors choline and folate reduces microbiome diversity and impairs intestinal structure in experimental mice while additionally impairing growth [35]. The role of essential amino acid metabolism in child undernutrition may also be mediated by the gut microbiome. Deficiency of angiotensin I-converting enzyme (peptidyl-dipeptidase A) 2 induces malnutrition-like enteropathy in mice through disturbed amino acid metabolism and gut dysbiosis [36]. These phenotypes are also transferred via fecal transplant to germ-free mice. However, dietary supplementation with the essential amino acid tryptophan restores intestinal function. The undernourished microbiome may not benefit from the supplementation of all micronutrients. A number of pathogenic microorganisms efficiently metabolize iron, which may worsen the infectious burden in the context of child undernutrition. In a trial of 6-month-old infants in a low-resource setting in Kenya, iron fortification led to unfavorable changes in the infant microbiome including increased abundance of pathogenic *E. coli* and other potentially pathogenic enterobacteriaceae in addition to elevated intestinal inflammation [37].

Targeting the Gut Microbiome in Child Malnutrition

Due to the expanding evidence for a causal role of the gut microbiome in child undernutrition, interventions targeting the gut microbiome pose potential as novel therapies to improve child growth.

Antibiotics
Antibiotics have demonstrated growth-promoting effects in livestock farming and experimental animals and have been associated with weight gain in children in high-income settings [38]. In addition to their effect on pathogen elimination, antibiotics alter the composition of the gut microbiome, which may plausibly alter its metabolic capacity. Large intervention studies of antibiotic therapy following treatment for SAM in Malawi, Niger, and Kenya have provided conflicting evidence for their benefits in recovering growth [11–13]. However, a large meta-analysis found that antibiotic use increased height by 0.04 cm/month and weight by 23.8 g/month in children in LMIC [10]. Mass administration of antibiotics in LMIC where undernutrition is prevalent also reduces child mortality [9]. However, the threat of antimicrobial resistance may provide a barrier to widespread antibiotic usage in the absence of clinical infection, without further evidence for widespread benefits on child mortality and growth.

Probiotics/Prebiotics
Prebiotics and probiotics provide an attractive approach to ameliorate the immature microbiome observed in child undernutrition; however, conclusive evidence for their benefit is lacking. A large trial of a combined probiotic/prebiotic intervention in children recovering from SAM in Malawi failed to improve mortality or growth outcomes [39]. However, a recent large trial of a combined

probiotic/prebiotic intervention to prevent new-born sepsis in India found a small increase in infant weight [40]. Probiotics have proven beneficial for reducing diarrhea in children following SAM, demonstrating a potential benefit to reduce the infectious burden of undernutrition [41]. Furthermore, a small study found that the well-studied probiotic *Lactobacillus rhamnosus* GG significantly reduced infections and improved nutritional status in children during treatment for undernutrition [42]. Future use of probiotics as therapies for child undernutrition must carefully consider probiotic strain-specificity and the ability of strains to colonize the dysfunctional intestine of undernourished children.

Microbiota-Directed Foods

Legumes contain resistant starch that is readily fermented by the gut microbiome in addition to being rich in protein, zinc, and other micronutrients. The fermentation of dietary fiber produces short-chain fatty acids and other metabolites, which play essential roles in maintaining the integrity of the intestinal barrier. A number of studies have begun to examine locally sourced legumes as sustainable interventions to prevent child undernutrition. Cowpeas and common beans have shown small but significant benefits in improving LAZ and EED biomarkers, respectively, in randomized trials in children in Malawi, which may be partially mediated through the fermentation of resistant starch by the microbiome [43, 44]. Recent data has provided promising evidence for the potential of 'microbiota-directed foods' to improve child growth. Gehrig and colleagues systematically selected, locally-sourced foods that specifically enhance microbiota 'maturity' in early life, showing that such microbiota-targeted foods enhance biomarkers of growth, bone formation, neurodevelopment and immune function in both experimental animals and undernourished children. Such microbiota-targeted therapies hence pose potential as promising alternatives to standard therapeutic and complementary foods in settings with high prevalence of child undernutrition [45].

Fecal Microbiome Transplantation

Fecal microbiome transplantation (FMT) has proven highly successful as treatment for individuals suffering from recurrent *C. difficile* infection and has displayed relatively beneficial effects in other chronic intestinal and metabolic disorders. FMT is yet untested in child undernutrition; however, an ongoing small pilot study of FMT in children with SAM whom are unresponsive to treatment will provide critical data on the feasibility and safety of this treatment for severe malnutrition (https://clinicaltrials.gov/ct2/show/NCT03087097).

Robertson

Conclusions

Research into the gut microbiome has led to novel therapies that have significantly improved both survival and quality of life in patients with chronic intestinal and metabolic disorders in high-income settings. This wealth of knowledge must now be applied with a global health perspective in LMIC in order to improve child mortality and undernutrition, both of which remain unacceptably high. Seventy-four out of every 1,000 live births results in death before 5 years of age in the WHO African Region alone, compared with 9 per 1,000 births in the WHO European Region. Almost 1 in 4 children globally are undernourished, leading to long-term growth and cognitive and health deficits. It is now evident that the gut microbiome plays a significant role in the metabolic and immune pathways that determine child growth, development, and tolerance to infectious disease. Expanding knowledge in this field suggests that if the gut microbiome is disturbed in early life, it may impair these growth and developmental processes, thereby contributing to high child mortality and undernutrition in LMIC.

Future research in this field must consider the role of the microbiome prenatally and even preconceptionally. As a large proportion of child undernutrition appears to occur in utero, the role of the maternal microbiome may plausibly influence offspring growth. Furthermore, with developments in sampling and sequencing technologies, it will be essential to consider not only the fecal microbiome but also the role of the microbiome in the upper gastrointestinal and other ecological niches within the body. Finally, with expanding knowledge from preclinical and observational studies, future research must begin to investigate microbiota-directed intervention strategies while carefully considering timing of intervention, infant baseline metabolic state, and mechanisms of action. In conjunction with other therapeutic approaches, microbiota-directed therapies pose real potential to reduce the mortality and morbidity associated with child undernutrition.

Funding Sources

RCR is in receipt of a fellowship from The Wellcome Trust (206455/Z/17/Z).

Disclosure Statement

The author declares no conflict of interest.

References

1 Black RE, Victora CG, Walker SP, et al; Maternal and Child Nutrition Study Group: Maternal and child undernutrition and overweight in low-income and middle-income countries. Lancet 2013; 382:427–451.

2 Adair LS, Fall CH, Osmond C, et al; COHORTS group: Associations of linear growth and relative weight gain during early life with adult health and human capital in countries of low and middle income: Findings from five birth cohort studies. Lancet 2013;382:525–534.

3 Bhutta ZA, Das JK, Rizvi A, et al; Lancet Nutrition Interventions Review Group; the Maternal and Child Nutrition Study Group: Evidence-based interventions for improvement of maternal and child nutrition: what can be done and at what cost? Lancet 2013;382:452–477.

4 Prendergast A, Kelly P: Enteropathies in the developing world: Neglected effects on global health. Am J Trop Med Hyg 2012;86:756–763.

5 MAL-ED Network Investigators: Childhood stunting in relation to the pre- and postnatal environment during the first 2 years of life: the MAL-ED longitudinal birth cohort study. PLoS Med 2017;14:e1002408.

6 MAL-ED Network Investigators: Relationship between growth and illness, enteropathogens and dietary intakes in the first 2 years of life: findings from the MAL-ED birth cohort study. BMJ Glob Health 2017;2:e000370.

7 Liu J, Platts-Mills JA, Juma J, et al: Use of quantitative molecular diagnostic methods to identify causes of diarrhoea in children: a reanalysis of the GEMS case-control study. Lancet 2016;388: 1291–1301.

8 Attia S, Versloot CJ, Voskuijl W, et al: Mortality in children with complicated severe acute malnutrition is related to intestinal and systemic inflammation: an observational cohort study. Am J Clin Nutr 2016;104:1441–1449.

9 Keenan JD, Bailey RL, West SK, et al; MORDOR Study Group: Azithromycin to reduce childhood mortality in sub-Saharan Africa. N Engl J Med 2018;378:1583–1592.

10 Gough EK, Moodie EE, Prendergast AJ, Jet al: The impact of antibiotics on growth in children in low and middle income countries: systematic review and meta-analysis of randomised controlled trials. BMJ 2014;348:g2267.

11 Trehan I, Goldbach HS, LaGrone LN, et al: Antibiotics as part of the management of severe acute malnutrition. N Engl J Med 2013;368:425–435.

12 Berkley JA, Ngari M, Thitiri J, et al: Daily co-trimoxazole prophylaxis to prevent mortality in children with complicated severe acute malnutrition: A multicentre, double-blind, randomised placebo-controlled trial. Lancet Glob Health 2016;4:e464–e473.

13 Isanaka S, Langendorf C, Berthé F, et al: Routine amoxicillin for uncomplicated severe acute malnutrition in children. N Engl J Med 2016;374: 444–453.

14 Robertson RC, Manges AR, Finlay BB, Prendergast AJ: The human microbiome and child growth – first 1000 days and beyond. Trends Microbiol 2019;27:131–147.

15 Aagaard K, Ma J, Antony KM, et al: The placenta harbors a unique microbiome. Sci Transl Med 2014;6:237ra65.

16 de Goffau MC, Lager S, Sovio U, et al. Human placenta has no microbiome but can contain potential pathogens. Nature 2019;572(7769);329–334.

17 Younge N, McCann JR, Ballard J, et al. Fetal exposure to the maternal microbiota in humans and mice. JCI Insight 2019;4(19).

18 Subramanian S, Huq S, Yatsunenko T, et al: Persistent gut microbiota immaturity in malnourished Bangladeshi children. Nature 2014;510: 417–421.

19 Prendergast AJ, Humphrey JH: The stunting syndrome in developing countries. Paediatr Int Child Health 2014;34:250–265.

20 Al Nabhani Z, Dulauroy S, Marques R, et al. A weaning reaction to microbiota is required for resistance to immunopathologies in the adult. Immunity 2019;50(5):1276–1288.

21 Vonaesch P, Morien E, Andrianonimiadana L, et al: Stunted childhood growth is associated with decompartmentalization of the gastrointestinal tract and overgrowth of oropharyngeal taxa. Proc Natl Acad Sci USA 2018;115:E8489–E8498.

22 Dinh DM, Ramadass B, Kattula D, Sarkar R, Braunstein P, Tai A, Wanke CA, Hassoun S, Kane AV, Naumova EN, Kang G, Ward HD: Longitudinal analysis of the intestinal microbiota in persistently stunted young children in South India. PLoS One 2016;11:e0155405.

23 Gough EK, Stephens DA, Moodie EE, Prendergast AJ, Stoltzfus RJ, Humphrey JH, Manges AR: Linear growth faltering in infants is associated with Acidaminococcus sp. and community-level changes in the gut microbiota. Microbiome 2015; 3:24.

24 Brown EM, Wlodarska M, Willing BP, et al: Diet and specific microbial exposure trigger features of environmental enteropathy in a novel murine model. Nat Commun 2015;6:7806.

25 Schwarzer M, Makki K, Storelli G, et al: Lactoba-cillus plantarum strain maintains growth of infant mice during chronic undernutrition. Science 2016;351:854–857.

26 Charbonneau MR, O'Donnell D, Blanton LV, et al: Sialylated milk oligosaccharides promote microbiota-dependent growth in models of infant undernutrition. Cell 2016;164:859–871.

27 Wagner VE, Dey N, Guruge J, et al: Effects of a gut pathobiont in a gnotobiotic mouse model of childhood undernutrition. Sci Transl Med 2016; 8:366ra164.

28 Kerac M, Bunn J, Chagaluka G, et al: Follow-up of post-discharge growth and mortality after treatment for severe acute malnutrition (FuSAM study): a prospective cohort study. PLoS One 2014;9:e96030.

29 Raman AS, Gehrig JL, Venkatesh S, et al. A sparse covarying unit that describes healthy and impaired human gut microbiota development. Science 2019;365(6449):pii:eaau4735.

30 Million M, Tidjani Alou M, Khelaifia S, et al: Increased gut redox and depletion of anaerobic and methanogenic prokaryotes in severe acute malnutrition. Sci Rep 2016;6:26051.

31 Smith MI, Yatsunenko T, Manary MJ, et al: Gut microbiomes of Malawian twin pairs discordant for kwashiorkor. Science 2013;339:548–554.

32 Blanton LV, Charbonneau MR, Salih T, et al: Gut bacteria that prevent growth impairments transmitted by microbiota from malnourished children. Science 2016;351.

33 Kau AL, Planer JD, Liu J, et al: Functional characterization of IgA-targeted bacterial taxa from undernourished Malawian children that produce diet-dependent enteropathy. Sci Transl Med 2015;7:276ra24.

34 Hibberd MC, Wu M, Rodionov DA, et al: The effects of micronutrient deficiencies on bacterial species from the human gut microbiota. Sci Transl Med 2017;9:pii:eaal4069.

35 Alves da Silva AV, de Castro Oliveira SB, Di Rienzi SC, et al: Murine methyl donor deficiency impairs early growth in association with dysmorphic small intestinal crypts and reduced gut microbial community diversity. Curr Dev Nutr 2019;3:nzy070.

36 Hashimoto T, Perlot T, Rehman A, et al: ACE2 links amino acid malnutrition to microbial ecology and intestinal inflammation. Nature 2012; 487:477–481.

37 Jaeggi T, Kortman GA, Moretti D, et al: Iron fortification adversely affects the gut microbiome, increases pathogen abundance and induces intestinal inflammation in Kenyan infants. Gut 2015; 64:731–742.

38 Bailey LC, Forrest CB, Zhang P, et al: Association of antibiotics in infancy with early childhood obesity. JAMA Pediatr 2014;168:1063–1069.

39 Kerac M, Bunn J, Seal A, et al: Probiotics and prebiotics for severe acute malnutrition (PRONUT study): a double-blind efficacy randomised controlled trial in Malawi. Lancet 2009;374:136–144.

40 Panigrahi P, Parida S, Nanda NC, et al: A randomized synbiotic trial to prevent sepsis among infants in rural India. Nature 2017;548:407–412.

41 Grenov B, Namusoke H, Lanyero B, et al: Effect of probiotics on diarrhea in children with severe acute malnutrition: a randomized controlled study in Uganda. J Pediatr Gastroenterol Nutr 2017;64:396–403.

42 Kara SS, Volkan B, Erten I: Lactobacillus rhamnosus GG can protect malnourished children. Benef Microbes 2019;1–8.

43 Agapova SE, Stephenson KB, Divala O, et al: Additional common bean in the diet of Malawian children does not affect linear growth, but reduces intestinal permeability. J Nutr 2018;148:267–274.

44 Stephenson KB, Agapova SE, Divala O, et al: Complementary feeding with cowpea reduces growth faltering in rural Malawian infants: a blind, randomized controlled clinical trial. Am J Clin Nutr 2017;106:1500–1507.

45 Gehrig JL, Venkatesh S, Chang HW, et al. Effects of microbiota-directed foods in gnotobiotic animals and undernourished children. Science 2019; 365(6449):pii:eaau4732.

Michaelsen KF, Neufeld LM, Prentice AM (eds): Global Landscape of Nutrition Challenges in
Infants and Children. Nestlé Nutr Inst Workshop Ser, vol 93, pp 145–151, (DOI: 10.1159/000503351)
Nestlé Nutrition Institute, Switzerland/S. Karger AG., Basel, © 2020

Intergenerational Influences on Child Development: An Epigenetic Perspective

Matt J. Silver

MRC Unit The Gambia at the London School of Tropical Medicine and Hygiene, London, UK

Abstract

The link between poor maternal nutrition and suboptimal outcomes in offspring is well established, but underlying mechanisms are not well understood. Modifications to the offspring epigenome are a plausible mechanism for the transmission of intergenerational signals that could extend to effects of paternal nutrition mediated by epigenetic modifications in sperm. The epigenome is extensively remodeled in the early embryo. Attention has therefore focused on the periconceptional period as a time when differences in parental nutrition might influence the establishment of epigenetic marks in offspring. So-called "natural experiments" in The Gambia and elsewhere have highlighted loci that may be especially sensitive to periconceptional nutrition, and some are associated with health-related outcomes in later life. There is speculation that some epigenetic signals could be transmitted across multiple generations, although this would require epigenetic marks to evade epigenetic reprogramming events at conception and in primordial germ cells, and evidence for this is lacking in humans. Effects on child development spanning one or more generations could impose an intergenerational "brake" on a child's growth potential, limiting, for example, the rate at which populations can escape from stunting.

© 2020 Nestlé Nutrition Institute, Switzerland/S. Karger AG, Basel

Epidemiological evidence indicates that suboptimal maternal nutrition is associated with a wide range of adverse outcomes in offspring throughout the life course, but underlying mechanisms are poorly understood [1]. Evidence from

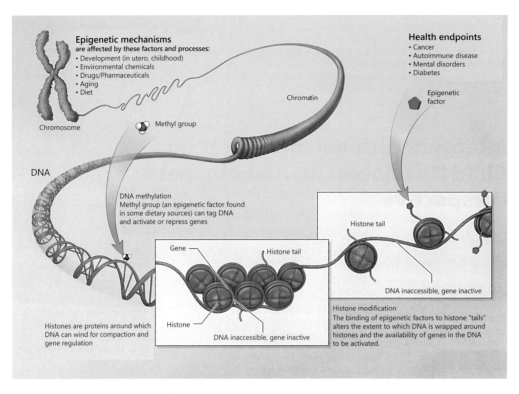

Fig. 1. Epigenetic mechanisms may mediate links between early environmental exposures and health outcomes in later life (Image courtesy of US National Institutes of Health).

animal models and some human data suggest that modifications to the developing offspring epigenome (Fig. 1) offer a plausible mediating mechanism since (i) they can be sensitive to the early environment in gestation; (ii) they can influence gene expression and have been associated with numerous metabolic and other traits; and (iii) there is the potential for intergenerational transmission of epigenetic signals [2]. However, the study of these effects in humans is challenging. Epigenetic marks are often tissue-specific, and it may be difficult or impossible to access a disease-specific tissue of interest. Furthermore, associations may be confounded by the influence of genetic variation. Finally, causal pathways are difficult to elucidate in observational studies, and even randomized experimental designs are prone to confounding due to reverse causation effects [3].

One widely studied epigenetic process involves the addition of methyl groups to DNA. DNA methylation (DNAm) marks are faithfully copied across cell divisions in mitosis and can influence gene expression without altering the underlying DNA sequence. DNAm plays a key role in several cellular processes including the establishment and maintenance of cellular identity, X-chromosome inactivation, and genomic imprinting. Importantly, DNAm marks are extensively remodeled in the very early embryo when maternal and paternal gametic methylation marks are erased in order to render embryonic cells into a totipotent state, ready to acquire tissue-specific marks at implantation, gastrulation, and beyond. Attention has therefore focused on the periconceptional period as a time when the establishment of epigenetic marks in offspring might be especially sensitive to differences in maternal (and potentially paternal) nutrition [4].

Nutrition plays a part in the establishment, maintenance, and erasure of DNAm marks through the action of one-carbon and 10–11 translocation enzyme-mediated pathways that rely on so-called "methyl donor" nutrients including folate and other B vitamins, choline, betaine, and vitamin C that are derived from our diets [5]. Robust evidence linking early nutrition to health-related phenotypic effects mediated by DNAm changes comes from the Agouti mouse model, with methyl donor-supplemented dams producing an excess of obese, metabolically dysfunctional offspring, driven by DNAm changes in a cryptic Agouti gene promoter [6]. Evidence of in utero nutrient-offspring DNAm associations in humans is rapidly accumulating, with diverse although sometimes inconsistent effects reported from both observational and randomized study designs investigating a range of nutrient exposures throughout gestation [7].

A major motivation for research in the field of human epigenetic epidemiology comes from so-called "natural experiments" that have shown intergenerational associations between parental or grandparental nutrition and offspring morbidity and mortality [8–11]. In these studies, individuals exposed to a range of early-life and peripubertal factors including famine, poor harvests, and exposure to Ramadan are compared to controls, with the period in early gestation often highlighted as a window of heightened sensitivity. However, few of these studies, some of which rely on historical data stretching back to the 19th century, have been able to look at epigenetic effects directly, with the notable exception of investigations relating to in utero famine exposure in the "Dutch Hunger Winter" [12].

A series of studies in The Gambia in sub-Saharan West Africa exploits another natural experiment whereby fluctuations in maternal energy balance and nutritional exposures show a distinct bimodal pattern corresponding to dry and rainy seasons. Season of birth has been linked to mortality in this population, with differential survival rates not manifesting until adolescence, suggesting the potential for an epigenetically-mediated effect of early-life adversity on later health [13]. Associations between *parental* season of birth and offspring anthropometry have also been observed [14]. Here, the discovery of an association with paternal season of birth is of particular interest since a patrilineal effect is most likely to be mediated through the father's sperm.

Progress has also been made in identifying the effects of Gambian seasonality on DNAm. We have shown, for example, that season of conception and levels of certain nutritional biomarkers in maternal blood plasma at conception predict DNAm in infants at a number of putative metastable epialleles – genomic regions where methylation is established in the early embryo [15–19]. Several of these loci have been associated with molecular traits and health outcomes including obesity, immune function, and cancer [17, 18, 20]. The link to obesity involves a variably methylated region of the proopiomelanocortin (POMC) gene that is involved in the regulation of appetite. Evidence that POMC methylation is established in early life, is associated with periconceptional environment, is stable thereafter, and is associated with POMC expression positions this locus as a strong candidate for mediating links between early-life nutrition and the regulation of bodyweight in later life in humans [18, 21].

This and related work in human nutritional epigenetics focus on the potential for DNAm changes to mediate "intergenerational" signals, that is, methylation changes that arise as a result of direct exposure of the embryo or fetus to maternal factors. Intergenerational epigenetic effects additionally encompass paternal and grandmaternal exposures, since germ cells that give rise to the current generation could have been exposed in utero (Fig. 2, dark grey-shaded areas).

There is currently a great deal of interest in the possibility that epigenetic signals might also be transmitted across multiple generations in so-called "transgenerational epigenetic inheritance," where subsequent generations have not been directly exposed (Fig. 2, light grey-shaded areas). Epidemiological evidence for putative transgenerational effects comes, for example, from the Swedish Överkalix and Uppsala studies that show an association between grand paternal exposure to poor nutrition and male grandchild all-cause mortality [8, 9]. However, there is skepticism that such observations could be mediated by epigenetic modifications since this would require epigenetic states to escape 2 waves of epigenetic reprogramming, the first at conception and the second during the development of primordial germ cells in gestation. Evidence for this is currently lacking in humans.

Despite this, efforts are ongoing to identify examples of transgenerational epigenetic inheritance in mammals, motivated in part by robust examples of this phenomenon in plants and lower animals. For example, transgenerational epigenetic mechanisms have been shown to mediate the inheritance of corn kernel colors in maize plants through the action of small interfering RNAs [22], and transgenerational epigenetic inheritance has also been observed to mediate the multigeneration effect of heat exposure in nematode worms, in this case through the action of histone modifications [23]. Work in mammals is focused on the mouse. Examples typically involve severe exposures such as postnatal trauma

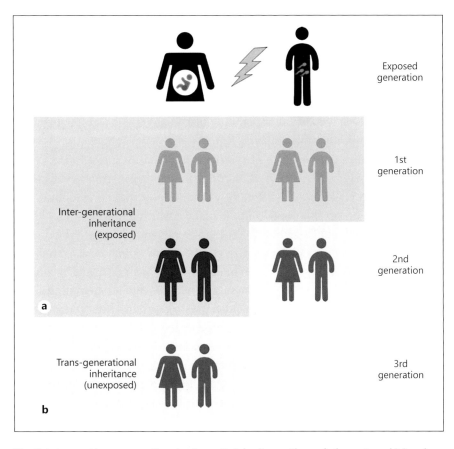

Fig. 2. Inter- and transgenerational epigenetic inheritance through the maternal (**a**) and paternal (**b**) lines.

and exposure to endocrine disruptors, leading to widespread metabolic or developmental pathologies, with regions of DNAm that escape reprogramming and sperm RNAs emerging as leading candidate epigenetic mechanisms [24–26].

Depending on the context, DNAm and other epigenetic changes that are driven by environmental exposures in early life or in preceding generations could be classified as epigenetic errors or as adaptations. The latter case is often referred to as *epigenetic programming* or as an example of a *predictive adaptive response* [27]. In the context of early maternal nutrition, we might speculate that DNAm or other epigenetic marks that are responsive to the periconceptional nutrition milieu could have evolved to sense the environment, record the information, and adapt the organism to its anticipated postnatal environment. Where there is a mismatch between pre- and postnatal environments, this would lead to maladaptation and potentially to disease. In this way, regions of epigenetic variability at a population level could provide a substrate for adaptation to rapidly changing environments in a manner not amenable to adaption through Darwinian genetic evolution that typically operates over much slower timescales [28]. Importantly, the evolution of such a mechanism would require that epigenetically variability at environmentally responsive loci is under genetic control. In support of this, evidence is emerging that increased variability at certain DNAm loci may be driven by genotype [20, 29, 30], suggesting that some intergenerational DNAm signals might fall within the *predictive adaptive response* paradigm.

In conclusion, a diverse range of epigenetic mechanisms might influence the growth and development of children. Nutritional and other environmental insults affecting parents could plausibly affect their children, potentially providing an "intergenerational brake" that would limit the rate at which individuals (and hence populations) can escape from the effects of an adverse family history. The possibility of longer-range effects spanning several generations cannot be ruled out, but currently lacks convincing evidence in humans. Either scenario would encourage a counsel of patience when judging the success of interventions attempting to enhance the growth of children through either pre- or postnatal dietary supplementation, since a proportional gain over several generations might be the best that can be expected. Furthermore, to the extent that epigenetic mechanisms may underlie predictive adaptive responses, where there is a mismatch between a child's early- and later-life nutritional experiences, a gradualist approach might offer the optimal trajectory for moving populations from nutritional poverty.

Disclosure Statement

The author declares no conflicts of interest. The author is supported by core funding to MRC Unit The Gambia from the UK MRC and UK Department for the International Development (DFID) under the MRC/DFID Concordat agreement (MC-A760-5QX00).

References

1 Barker DJ, Thornburg KL: The Obstetric origins of health for a lifetime. Clin Obstet Gynecol 2013; 56:511–519.

2 Bianco-Miotto T, Craig JM, Gasser YP, et al: Epigenetics and DOHaD: from basics to birth and beyond. J Dev Orig Health Dis 2017;8:513–519.

3 Relton CL, Davey Smith G: Is epidemiology ready for epigenetics? Int J Epidemiol 2012;41:5–9.

4 Fleming TP, Watkins AJ, Velazquez MA, et al: Origins of lifetime health around the time of conception: causes and consequences. Lancet 2018; 391:1842–1852.

5 Dominguez-Salas P, Cox SE, Prentice AM, et al: Maternal nutritional status, C(1) metabolism and offspring DNA methylation: A review of current evidence in human subjects. Proc Nutr Soc 2012; 71:154–165.

6 Waterland RA, Jirtle RL: Transposable elements: targets for early nutritional effects on epigenetic gene regulation. Mol Cell Biol 2003;23:5293–5300.

7 James P, Sajjadi S, Tomar AS, et al: Candidate genes linking maternal nutrient exposure to offspring health via DNA methylation: a review of existing evidence in humans with specific focus on one-carbon metabolism. Int J Epidemiol 2018; 47: 1910–1937.

8 Pembrey ME, Bygren LO, Kaati G, et al: Sex-specific, male-line transgenerational responses in humans. Eur J Hum Genet 2006;14:159–166.

9 Vågerö D, Pinger PR, Aronsson V, van den Berg GJ: Paternal grandfather's access to food predicts all-cause and cancer mortality in grandsons. Nat Commun 2018;9:5124.

10 Lumey LH, Stein AD, Susser E: Prenatal famine and adult health. Annu Rev Public Health 2011; 32:237–262.

11 Schoeps A, van Ewijk R, Kynast-Wolf G, et al: Ramadan exposure in utero and child mortality in Burkina Faso: Analysis of a population-based cohort including 41,025 children. Am J Epidemiol 2018;187:2085–2092.

12 Tobi EW, Goeman JJ, Monajemi R, et al: DNA methylation signatures link prenatal famine exposure to growth and metabolism. Nat Commun 2014;5:5592.

13 Moore SE, Cole TJ, Collinson AC, et al: Prenatal or early postnatal events predict infectious deaths in young adulthood in rural Africa. Int J Epidemiol 1999;28:1088–1095.

14 Eriksen KG, Radford EJ, Silver MJ, et al: Influence of intergenerational in utero parental energy and nutrient restriction on offspring growth in rural Gambia. FASEB J 2017;31:4928–4934.

15 Waterland RA, Kellermayer R, Laritsky E, et al: Season of conception in rural Gambia affects DNA methylation at putative human metastable epialleles. PLoS Genet 2010;6:e1001252.

16 Dominguez-Salas P, Moore SE, Baker MS, et al: Maternal nutrition at conception modulates DNA methylation of human metastable epialleles. Nat Commun 2014;5:3746.

17 Silver MJ, Kessler NJ, Hennig BJ, et al: Independent genomewide screens identify the tumor suppressor VTRNA2-1 as a human epiallele responsive to periconceptional environment. Genome Biol 2015;16:118.

18 Kühnen P, Handke D, Waterland RA, et al: Inter-individual variation in DNA methylation at a putative POMC metastable epiallele is associated with obesity. Cell Metab 2016;24:502–509.

19 Kessler NJ, Waterland RA, Prentice AM, Silver MJ: Establishment of environmentally sensitive DNA methylation states in the very early human embryo. Sci Adv 2018;4:eaat2624.

20 Van Baak TE, Coarfa C, Dugué PA, et al: Epigenetic supersimilarity of monozygotic twin pairs. Genome Biol 2018;19:2.

21 Kuehnen P, Mischke M, Wiegand S, et al: An alu element-associated hypermethylation variant of the POMC gene is associated with childhood obesity. PLoS Genet 2012;8:e1002543.

22 Erhard KF, Parkinson SE, Gross SM, et al: Maize RNA polymerase IV defines trans-generational epigenetic variation. Plant Cell 2013;25:808–819.

23 Klosin A, Casas E, Hidalgo-Carcedo C, et al: Transgenerational transmission of environmental information in C. elegans. Science 2017;356: 320–323.

24 Gapp K, van Steenwyk G, Germain PL, et al: Alterations in sperm long RNA contribute to the epigenetic inheritance of the effects of postnatal trauma. Mol Psychiatry 2018.

25 Guerrero-Bosagna C, Covert TR, Haque MM, et al: Epigenetic transgenerational inheritance of vinclozolin induced mouse adult onset disease and associated sperm epigenome biomarkers. Reprod Toxicol 2012;34:694–707.

26 Chen Q, Yan W, Duan E: Epigenetic inheritance of acquired traits through sperm RNAs and sperm RNA modifications. Nat Rev Genet 2016; 17:733–743.

27 Low FM, Gluckman PD, Hanson MA: Developmental plasticity, epigenetics and human health. Evol Biol 2012;39:650–665.

28 Feinberg AP, Irizarry RA: Stochastic epigenetic variation as a driving force of development, evolutionary adaptation, and disease. Proc Natl Acad Sci 2010;107(suppl 1):1757–1764.

29 Plongthongkum N, van Eijk KR, de Jong S, et al: Characterization of Genome-Methylome Interactions in 22 Nuclear Pedigrees. PLoS One 2014; 9:e99313.

30 Ek WE, Rask-Andersen M, Karlsson T, et al: Genetic variants influencing phenotypic variance heterogeneity. Hum Mol Genet 2018;27:799–810.

Michaelsen KF, Neufeld LM, Prentice AM (eds): Global Landscape of Nutrition Challenges in Infants and Children. Nestlé Nutr Inst Workshop Ser, vol 93, pp 153–166, (DOI: 10.1159/000503350)
Nestlé Nutrition Institute, Switzerland/S. Karger AG., Basel, © 2020

Summarizing the Child Growth and Diarrhea Findings of the Water, Sanitation, and Hygiene Benefits and Sanitation Hygiene Infant Nutrition Efficacy Trials

Rachel R. Makasi[a] · Jean H. Humphrey[a, b]

[a] Zvitambo Institute for Maternal and Child Health Research, Harare, Zimbabwe; [b] Department of International Health, Johns Hopkins Bloomberg School of Public Health, Baltimore, MD, USA

Abstract

Stunting is a prevalent form of child undernutrition and is associated with lifelong adverse health outcomes and loss of human capital. The Water, Sanitation, and Hygiene (WASH) Benefits (Bangladesh and Kenya) and Sanitation Hygiene Infant Nutrition Efficacy (SHINE; Zimbabwe) trials were conducted to test the independent and combined effects of improved household WASH (improved pit latrine, handwashing station not connected to a water source, point-of-use water chlorination) and improved infant and young child feeding (IYCF, complementary feeding counseling and daily small-quantity lipid nutrient supplement) on child linear growth. Together the trials enrolled >19,000 women during pregnancy and measured >15,000 of their children at 18 months (SHINE) or 24 months (WASH Benefits trials) of age. Throughout the 3 trials, the IYCF intervention increased mean length-for-age Z-score by 0.13–0.26. None of the WASH interventions had any effect on linear growth among any of the study populations. This lack of effect is most likely because the household-level elementary WASH interventions employed in the trials were not effective enough in reducing

All trials received funding from the Bill and Melinda Gates Foundation (OPPGD759) for WASH Benefits Bangladesh and Kenya trials and (OPP1021542 and OPP1143707) for SHINE trial. WASH Benefits Kenya also received funding from United States Agency for International Development (AID-0AA-F-13-00040). SHINE also received funding from the United Kingdom Department for International Development (DFID/UKAID); Wellcome Trust (093768/Z/10/Z and 108065/Z/15/Z) and the Swiss Agency for Development and Cooperation.

enteropathogen exposure to facilitate linear growth. Consensus papers of the trials recommend identification and implementation of "transformative WASH" – interventions that radically reduce fecal exposure – to be made available to rural low-income populations.

Introduction

Globally, 22% (149 million) of the world's under-5 children are stunted, having a height-for-age Z-score below –2.0 [1]. About 20% of stunting occurs in utero [2], and the remainder occurs by 18–24 months of age [3]. Children who are stunted by 2–3 years of age are more likely to die before their fifth birthday, attend fewer years of school, earn less money as adults, and develop metabolic diseases like diabetes, obesity, and hypertension [4]. Children of women who were stunted as young children are at higher risk of stunting themselves, perpetuating the problems into future generations [4].

Stunting is surprisingly recalcitrant to interventions to improve dietary intake during the first 2 years of life. A recent systematic review concluded that, on average, complementary feeding interventions increase length-for-age Z-score (LAZ) by 0.11, which is only 5–10% of the deficit experienced by Asian and African children [5].

UNICEF's 1990 Framework of Undernutrition attributes stunting and other forms of undernutrition to a composite of multiple proximal and distal factors [6]. Chief among these is unsafe water, lack of sanitation, and poor personal hygiene (Water, Sanitation, and Hygiene [WASH]), primarily for its role in diarrheal disease. We have hypothesized that the adverse effects of poor WASH on growth may be mediated through environmental enteric dysfunction (EED) in addition to diarrhea [7]. EED is a subclinical condition of the small intestine characterized by reduced surface area for nutrient absorption, inflammation, and permeability, which facilitates translocation of microbes into local lymph nodes and the systemic circulation, thereby triggering chronic inflammation [8]. Dozens of papers from numerous low-income countries suggest that EED is virtually ubiquitous among people living in conditions of poverty [7]. Many of these studies suggest that exposure to fecal contamination is the cause of EED. Accordingly, we further hypothesized that minimizing fecal exposure by young children through an intensive WASH intervention would reduce EED and diarrhea, and improve linear growth, and that the beneficial effects of WASH on growth would be additive to those of improved complementary feeding [9].

Three trials were recently published, which tested the independent and combined effects of improving household WASH and improving infant diet on child growth and diarrhea: WASH Benefits Bangladesh [10], WASH Benefits Kenya [11], and the Sanitation Hygiene Infant Nutrition Efficacy (SHINE) [12] trial in Zimbabwe. In addition to the primary findings, many secondary findings and substudy analyses from these trials have been published [13–19]. In this paper, we summarize the findings of the 3 trials on child LAZ, weight-for-height Z-score, head circumference-for-age Z-score (HCZ), and 7-day prevalence of diarrhea.

Methods

All 3 trials:
- Used a cluster-randomized design.
- Enrolled women during pregnancy and then followed their children to 18 months (SHINE) or 24 months (WASH Benefits trials) of age.
- Delivered the WASH interventions to the enrolled woman's household (or compound comprising about 2 households in Bangladesh) and the Nutrition interventions to the index child born to the enrolled woman.
- Delivered behavior change communication (BCC) based on published behavior change models during home visits by people employed from the study areas.
- Developed BCC based on years of formative work and iterative piloting and designed it based on published behavior change models to include participatory, engaging activities which elicited key emotions known to trigger promoted behaviors.
- Provided hardware and commodities free of charge (chlorine, soap, latrines, small-quantity lipid-based nutrient supplement [SQ-LNS]), so that cost or limited access would not constrain use.
- Measured outcomes by trained research staff employed by the studies who were regularly standardized in taking anthropometric measures of children; all 3 trials used the WHO definition for diarrhea (3 or more loose or watery stools in 24 h) and the same recall period (7 days).
- Were not masked to intervention assignment, given the nature of the interventions.
- Published statistical analysis plans before breaking code and analyzed data at intention-to-treat regardless of adherence.
- Were registered at ClinicalTrials.gov, were approved by local and international IRBs, obtained participant written informed consent, and convened data safety and monitoring committees.
  Methods that were specific to the individual trials are described below.

WASH Benefits Bangladesh
Between May 31, 2012, and July 7, 2013, the WASH Benefits Bangladesh trial enrolled 5,551 pregnant women, forming them into 720 clusters that were then randomly allocated to 1 of 7 treatment arms. Randomization was geographically pair-matched in blocks of 8 clusters. Interventions were delivered by field workers who visited households an average of 6 times per month (once-twice weekly). The 7 treatment arms were:
- *Point-of-use drinking water treatment (Water):* provision of a water storage container and regular delivery of chlorine tablets, plus BCC to promote treatment of all drinking water, especially that given to children.

- *Household sanitation (Sanitation):* provision of a pour-flush improved latrine in the compound, a dedicated tool for removing feces from the living area ("sani-scoop"), and a child potty, plus BCC to promote use of the latrine by all members of the family for all episodes of defecation.
- *Handwashing:* provision of 2 handwashing stations and regular delivery of soap plus BCC promoting handwashing with soap after defecation and before food preparation.
- *Nutrition:* provision of 20 g/day SQ-LNS for children from 6 to 24 months of age, plus BCC promoting dietary diversity and adequacy during complementary feeding.
- *WASH:* all interventions included in the water treatment, sanitation, and handwashing treatment groups delivered concurrently.
- *WASH + Nutrition:* all interventions included in the WASH and Nutrition arms delivered concurrently.
- *Control:* a double-sized group to optimize statistical power; control participants did not receive intervention visits, being visited only for outcome measurement.

Outcome Measurement
Women and children were followed up at 1 and 2 years after beginning the interventions when infants were a median age of 9 (IQR 8–10) months and 22 (IQR 21–24) months, respectively. At these visits, intervention adherence, prevalence of child diarrhea during the previous 7 days, and child length, weight, and head circumference were measured.

WASH Benefits Kenya
Between November 27, 2012, and May 21, 2014, the WASH Benefits Kenya trial enrolled 8,246 pregnant women, forming them into 702 clusters which were then randomized to 7 intervention arms that were similar to those implemented in WASH Benefits Bangladesh with these differences: the Water treatment delivered liquid chlorine through chlorine dispensers installed at the points of water collection within the clusters randomized to Water, WASH, and WASH + Nutrition. A bottle of chlorine was also provided to these study households for use when water was obtained from a source that did not have a chlorine dispenser. Improved latrines were achieved by installing a plastic slab with a tight-fitting lid or by building a new improved latrine in households without a latrine. Handwashing stations were tippy taps with 2 containers – one with soapy water achieved by regularly adding chunks of soap to the water and the other with rinse water. WASH Benefits Kenya had 2 control arms: 1 in which mid-upper-arm circumference was measured in children during household visits at the same intervals as other intervention groups; the other in which households were visited only for research outcomes. Intervention visits occurred monthly.

Outcome Measurement
Women and children were followed up at 1 and 2 years after beginning the interventions when infants were a median age of 12 (range 2–18) months and 25 (range 16–31) months, respectively. At these visits, intervention adherence, prevalence of child diarrhea during the previous 7 days, and child length, weight, and head circumference were measured.

Sanitation Hygiene Infant Nutrition Efficacy
SHINE was a 2×2 factorial trial. Clusters were defined as the catchment area of 1–4 village health workers (VHWs) employed by the Zimbabwe Ministry of Health and Child

Care (MoHCC) and were randomized prior to enrollment to 1 of 4 treatment groups using a constrained randomization technique achieved balance across arms for 14 variables related to geography, demography, water access, and sanitation coverage. Between November 22, 2012, and March 27, 2015, 5,280 women living in the study area who became pregnant during the enrollment period were identified by prospective pregnancy surveillance and enrolled. Interventions were delivered by VHWs during visits at monthly intervals from recruitment to 12 months postpartum; between 13 and 18 months postpartum, VHWs continued monthly visits providing routine MoHCC care, and, in active arms, delivering intervention commodities and informally encouraging participants to practice treatment-arm-specific behaviors. HIV prevalence among antenatal women is 15% in Zimbabwe; because infant HIV infection and even exposure to maternal HIV infection strongly influence birth outcomes, growth, and development, the trial investigators prespecified that all outcomes would be stratified by maternal HIV status.

The 4 treatment groups were:

- Standard of Care (SOC): promotion of exclusive breastfeeding to 6 months and uptake of primary health care services from the MoHCC clinic.
- WASH: All SOC messages *plus*: (1) safe disposal of feces; (2) handwashing with soap at key times; (3) protection of infants from geophagia and animal feces ingestion; (4) chlorination of drinking water especially for infant; and (5) hygienic preparation of complementary food. A ventilated improved pit latrine was constructed at the household; 2 tippy tap handwashing stations were installed; a plastic mat and play yard (North States, Minneapolis, MN, USA) were delivered at 2 and 6 months postpartum, respectively; and soap and chlorine solutions were delivered monthly from –24 gestational weeks and 4 months postpartum, respectively.
- Infant and young child feeding (IYCF) Nutrition: All SOC messages *plus*: (1) overview of the role of nutrition for child growth and development; (2) feeding nutrient-dense food and 20 g SQ-LNS daily from 6 to 18 months, which was delivered to the home monthly; (3) processing locally available foods to facilitate mastication and swallowing; (4) feeding during illness; and (5) dietary diversity.
- WASH + IYCF: All SOC, WASH, and IYCF interventions.

Outcome data collection

At baseline (–14 weeks gestation), mothers were tested for HIV (rapid test algorithm); HIV-positive women were urged to seek immediate antenatal care for PMTCT interventions. Follow-up data were collected at 32 weeks of gestation and at infant ages 1, 3, 6, 12, and 18 months. At these visits, intervention adherence, prevalence of child diarrhea during the previous 7 days, and child length, weight, and head circumference were measured.

Findings

Together, the 3 trials enrolled >19,000 pregnant women (Table 1) and measured growth in >15,000 infants at 18–24 months of age (Table 2). Mothers in Zimbabwe had about 3 more years of schooling compared to those in Bangladesh and Kenya. Electricity was common among households in the Bangladesh, but not in the African sites; having a cement floor was more common in Zimbabwe

Table 1. Maternal and household baseline characteristics of the WASH Benefits Bangladesh, WASH Benefits Kenya, and SHINE study populations

Baseline characteristics	WASH Benefits Bangladesh n = 5,551 women	WASH Benefits Kenya n = 8,246 women	SHINE n = 5,280 women enrolled including 334 HIV-unknown HIV-negative n = 4,162[1]	HIV-positive n = 784[2]
Maternal, χ (SD)				
Age, years	24 (5)	26 (6)	26 (7)	29 (6)
Completed years of schooling	6 (3)	See note[3]	10 (2)	9 (2)
Household				
Number of occupants, χ (SD)	5 (2)[4]	8 (5)	5 (2)	5 (2)
Has a cement floor, %	11	6	52	57
Has electricity from power grid, %	59	7	3	3
Sanitation, %				
Household adult members who openly defecate	6	5	49	54
Own a latrine	54	82	36	33
Water				
Main source of drinking water is improved, %	74	74	62	59
Treat drinking water to make it safer, %	0	10	12	11
One-way walk time to fetch water, min, χ (SD)	See note[5]	11 (12)	20 (106)[6]	16 (24)[6]
Hygiene, %				
Hand-washing station at household with water and soap	2	10	<1	<1
Food Security, %				
Household is food insecure	31[7]	11[7]	20[8]	27[8]

[1] 3,902 women provided baseline data. Maternal and household data collected about 2 weeks after consent; this gap created opportunity for loss to follow-up between consent and baseline.
[2] 773 women provided baseline data. Maternal and household data collected about 2 weeks after consent; this gap created opportunity for loss to follow-up between consent and baseline.
[3] Data presented as proportion of women who completed primary school, which was 47%.
[4] Value is number of people per compound; there were an average of 2 households per compound.
[5] In Bangladesh, nearly all households had a water pipe stand within their compound.
[6] Distribution was highly skewed to high. Median (IQR) distance was 10 (5–20) min.
[7] Assessed by household food insecurity access scale.
[8] Assessed as proportion with coping strategy index >10.

than Bangladesh or Kenya. At baseline, open defecation by adult household members was much more common in Zimbabwe (50%) compared to Kenya and Bangladesh (5–6%); treating water to make it safer was uncommon in all 3 populations. Access to water differed substantially across study sites: in Bangladesh, the majority of homesteads had a pipe stand on the compound, while in Kenya and Zimbabwe, mean one-way walk time to fetch water was 11 and 20 min, respectively (distance to water was highly skewed in Zimbabwe: median walk time was 10 min). The main source of drinking water was unimproved for 40% of

Table 2. Effect of WASH, combined WASH, nutrition, and combined nutrition plus WASH on infant LAZ , WHZ, and HCZ after 2 years of intervention exposure in WASH Benefits trials and at 18 months of age in SHINE trial

WASH Benefits

Group	Bangladesh n	mean (SD)	difference vs. control	Kenya n	mean (SD)	difference vs. control
LAZ						
Control	1,103	−1.79 (1.01)		1,535	−1.54 (1.11)	
Water	595	−1.86 (1.07)	−0.06 (−0.18, 0.05)	719	−1.58 (1.08)	−0.04 (−0.15 to 0.08)
Sanitation	579	−1.80 (1.07)	−0.02 (−0.14 to 0.09)	744	−1.61 (1.13)	−0.06 (−0.18 to 0.05)
Handwashing	570	−1.85 (0.99)	−0.07 (−0.18 to 0.04)	700	−1.60 (1.06)	−0.04 (−0.16 to 0.07)
WASH	579	−1.76 (1.01)	0.02 (−0.09 to 0.19)	719	−1.59 (1.05)	−0.03 (−0.14 to 0.08)
Nutrition	567	−1.53 (1.05)	0.25 (0.15 to 0.36)	695	−1.44 (1.11)	0.13 (0.01 to 0.25)
WASH + nutrition	591	−1.67 (1.01)	0.13 (0.02 to 0.24)	760	−1.39 (1.05)	0.16 (0.05 to 0.27)
WHZ						
Control	1,104	−0.88 (0.93)		1,536	0.11 (0.94)	
Water	596	−0.92 (0.97)	−0.04 (−0.14 to 0.05)	719	0.14 (0.95)	0.04 (−0.06 to 0.13)
Sanitation	580	−0.85 (0.95)	0.01 (−0.09 to 0.11)	740	0.05 (0.97)	−0.05 (−0.14 to 0.05)
Handwashing	570	−0.86 (0.94)	0.00 (−0.11 to 0.12)	700	0.09 (0.93)	−0.02 (−0.11 to 0.06)

Zimbabwe-SHINE

Group	HIV-unexposed n	mean (SD)	difference vs. control	HIV-exposed n	mean (SD)	difference vs. control
LAZ						
Standard of care	878	−1.57 (1.08)		145	−2.00 (1.20)	
IYCF	891	−1.47 (1.06)		146	−1.73 (1.10)	
WASH	914	−1.61 (1.01)		184	−1.97 (1.08)	
IYCF + WASH	988	−1.41 (1.06)		190	−1.73 (1.14)	
Non-IYCF	1,792	−1.44 (1.06)		329	−1.99 (1.13)	
IYCF	1,879	−1.59 (1.08)	0.16 (0.08 to 0.23)	336	−1.73 (1.12)	0.26 (0.09 to 0.43)
Non-WASH	1,769	−1.52 (1.07)		291	−1.87 (1.16)	
WASH	1,902	−1.50 (1.07)	0.02 (−0.06 to 0.09)	374	−1.85 (1.12)	0.01 (−0.16 to 0.18)
WHZ						
Control	875	0.05 (1.07)		146	−0.05 (1.07)	
IYCF	888	0.06 (1.11)		147	−0.16 (1.08)	
WASH	907	−0.01 (1.04)		181	−0.04 (1.12)	
IYCF + WASH	982	0.11 (1.04)		189	−0.11 (1.10)	

Table 2. Continued

Group	WASH Benefits						Group	Zimbabwe-SHINE					
	Bangladesh			Kenya				HIV-unexposed			HIV-exposed		
	n	mean (SD)	difference vs. control	n	mean (SD)	difference vs. control		n	mean (SD)	difference vs. control	n	mean (SD)	difference vs. control
WASH	580	-0.88 (1.01)	0.00 (-0.10 to 0.11)	714	0.08 (0.92)	-0.02 (-0.10 to 0.07)	Non-IYCF	1,782	0.02 (1.05)		327	-0.05 (1.10)	
Nutrition	567	-0.71 (1.00)	0.15 (0.04 to 0.26)	695	0.14 (0.92)	0.04 (-0.05 to 0.14)	IYCF	1,870	0.09 (1.07)	0.08 (0.00 to 0.15)	336	-0.13 (1.09)	-0.09 (-0.27 to 0.09)
WASH + nutrition	591	-0.79 (0.94)	0.09 (0.00 to 0.18)	762	0.18 (0.90)	0.09 (0.00 to 0.19)	Non-WASH	1,763	0.06 (1.09)		293	-0.10 (1.08)	
							WASH	1,889	0.05 (1.04)	-0.01 (-0.08 to 0.07)	372	-0.08 (1.11)	0.03 (-0.15 to 0.18)
HCZ													
Control	1,118	-1.61 (0.94)		1,545	-0.27 (1.02)		Control	872	-0.26 (1.08)		146	-0.55 (1.08)	
Water	594	-1.63 (0.91)	-0.04 (-0.14 to 0.06)	727	-0.27 (1.03)	0.02 (-0.08 to 0.12)	IYCF	885	-0.23 (1.07)		147	-0.51 (1.09)	
Sanitation	584	-1.61 (0.86)	-0.01 (-0.10 to 0.09)	745	-0.27 (1.04)	0.01 (-0.09 to 0.11)	WASH	906	-0.27 (1.09)		182	-0.53 (1.15)	
Handwashing	571	-1.56 (0.93)	0.05 (-0.06 to 0.15)	705	-0.29 (0.99)	0.00 (-0.10 to 0.10)	IYCF + WASH	983	-0.16 (1.06)		189	-0.38 (1.14)	
WASH	584	-1.59 (0.91)	0.03 (-0.07 to 0.12)	729	-0.30 (0.96)	-0.03 (-0.12 to 0.06)	Non-IYCF	1,778	-0.26 (1.08)		328	-0.54 (1.12)	
Nutrition	570	-1.45 (0.94)	0.16 (0.04 to 0.27)	695	-0.23 (0.99)	0.05 (-0.05 to 0.15)	IYCF	1,868	-0.19 (1.06)	0.07 (0.00 to 0.14)	336	-0.44 (1.12)	0.10 (-0.07 to 0.27)
WASH + nutrition	590	-1.51 (0.90)	0.11 (0.01 to 0.20)	763	-0.22 (0.99)	0.05 (-0.04 to 0.15)	Non-WASH	1,757	-0.24 (1.07)		293	-0.53 (1.09)	
							WASH	1,889	-0.21 (1.08)	0.03 (-0.04 to 0.10)	371	-0.46 (1.14)	0.07 (-0.10 to 0.24)

WASH, Water, Sanitation, and Hygiene; LAZ, length-for-age Z-score; WHZ, weight-for-height Z-score; HCZ, head circumference-for-age Z-score; SHINE, Sanitation Hygiene Infant Nutrition Efficacy; IYCF, infant and young child feeding.

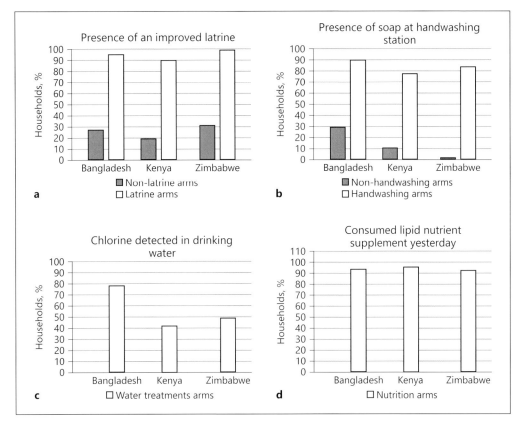

Fig. 1. Indicators of fidelity of intervention delivery and uptake of promoted behaviors 1 year after interventions began in Bangladesh and Kenya WASH Benefits trials and at 12 months of infant age in Zimbabwe SHINE trial.

Zimbabwean households compared to 25% of those in Bangladesh and Kenya. None of the study populations were experiencing famine conditions, while these studies were being conducted: across all 3 populations, 70–80% of household had enough food to satisfy hunger.

High fidelity of intervention delivery and good-to-high uptake of promoted behaviors resulted in substantial contrast between intervention and nonintervention arms for key indicators of environmental hygiene and infant diet. Figure 1 illustrates 4 key indicators at 1 year after interventions began in the WASH Benefits trials and at 12 months of infant age in the SHINE trial. In Bangladesh, Kenya, and Zimbabwe, respectively, 95, 90, and 99% of the households in sanitation-including arms had an improved latrine (Fig. 1a); 90, 78, and 84% of the households in arms including handwashing had soap or rubbing agent present at the handwashing station (Fig. 1b); and 80, 43, and ~50% of the households in arms including water treatment had detectable chlorine (Fig. 1c). In households randomized to infant nutrition, 94, 96, and 93% of infants in Bangladesh, Kenya, and Zimbabwe had consumed SQ-LNS on the previous day (Fig. 1d).

Among children in the control groups of the trials, mean LAZ of children at 18–24 months of age ranged from –1.54 in Kenya to –1.59 among children born to HIV-negative mothers in Zimbabwe, –1.79 in Bangladesh, and –2.00 among children born to HIV-positive mothers in Zimbabwe (Table 2). The corresponding proportions of these children who were stunted were 31, 33, 41, and 50%. These statistics can be compared to global estimates of stunting among children in the 24- to 35-month age-group of 29.4% (calculated for this age-group from UNICEF Malnutrition Rates, 2018, https://data.unicef.org/topic/nutrition/malnutrition/). Thus, the study populations experienced a level of stunting similar or higher to that of the average child in the world.

The IYCF intervention significantly improved LAZ and reduced stunting in all 3 trials. After 2 years of intervention exposure in Bangladesh, mean LAZ was 0.25 (0.15–0.36) and 0.13 (0.02–0.24) higher in the Nutrition only and WASH + Nutrition arms, respectively, compared to the control arm. These increases in LAZ corresponded to reductions in the proportion stunted from 41 to 33% (20% relative reduction) for the Nutrition-only arm and to 37% (10% relative reduction) for the Nutrition + WASH arm. Similarly, in Kenya, mean LAZ was 0.13 (0.01–0.25) and 0.16 (0.05–0.27) higher in the Nutrition and WASH + Nutrition arms, respectively, compared to the control arm after 2 years of intervention. These increases corresponded to a relative 7% reduction in stunting in the Nutrition arm (31–29%) and a relative 13% reduction in stunting in the Nutrition + WASH arm (31–27%). In SHINE, the IYCF intervention increased LAZ at 18 months of age by 0.16 (0.08–0.23) and 0.26 (0.09–0.43) among HIV-unexposed and HIV-exposed children, respectively. These increases corresponded to a relative 21% reduction in stunting among HIV-unexposed children (35–27%) and a relative 19% reduction in stunting among HIV-exposed children (50–40%). Overall, the magnitude of effect of the nutrition interventions on LAZ in these 3 trials was consistent with reports over several decades in the nutrition literature [5, 20, 21]. The impact of the nutrition interventions on linear growth was similar when the nutrition intervention was given alone compared to given concurrently with a WASH intervention.

The IYCF interventions also significantly improved mean weight-for-height Z-score by 0.08–0.15 in some comparisons: Bangladesh (Nutrition and Nutrition + WASH each compared to Control); Kenya (Nutrition + WASH compared to Control); and Zimbabwe (HIV-unexposed, IYCF compared to Non-IYCF).

Similar to other studies that included children from both South Asian and sub-Saharan African [22], head circumference was markedly smaller among Bangladeshi compared to Kenyan or Zimbabwean children: among control children at 18–24 months, mean HCZ was –1.67 (0.94) in Bangladesh, compared to

Table 3. Intervention effects on 7-day diarrhea prevalence

		Prevalence, %	Absolute difference (95% CI)	Relative difference (95% CI)
WASH Benefits Bangladesh	Control	5.7	Reference	Reference
	Water	4.9	−0.6 (−1.9 to +0.6)	0.89 (0.70 to 1.13)
	Sanitation	3.5	−2.2 (−3.4 to −1.0)	0.61 (0.46 to 0.81)
	Handwashing	3.5	−2.3 (−3.4 to −1.1)	0.60 (0.45 to 0.80)
	WASH	3.9	−1.7 (−2.9 to −0.6)	0.69 (0.53 to 0.90)
	Nutrition	3.5	−2.0 (−3.1 to −0.8)	0.64 (0.49 to 0.85)
	WASH + Nutrition	3.5	−2.2 (−3.3 to −1.0)	0.62 (0.47 to 0.81)
WASH Benefits Kenya	Control	27.1	Reference	Reference
	Water	27.7	+0.7 (−2.3 to +3.6)	1.02 (0.92 to 1.14)
	Sanitation	26.5	−0.3 (−3.3 to +2.6)	0.99 (0.88 to 1.10)
	Handwashing	26.1	−0.6 (−3.5 to +2.3)	0.98 (0.87 to 1.09)
	WASH	26.1	−1.2 (−4.1 to +1.7)	0.96 (0.86 to 1.07)
	Nutrition	25.5	−1.0 (−4.0 to +2.0)	0.96 (0.86 to 1.08)
	WASH + Nutrition	28.4	+1.2 (−1.7 to +4.1)	1.05 (0.94 to 1.16)
SHINE Infants of HIV-negative women	No IYCF	9.9	Reference	Reference
	IYCF	9.4	−0.5 (−0.9 to +2.9)	0.95 (0.77 to 1.16)
	No WASH	8.4	Reference	Reference
	WASH	10.7	+ 2.3 (+1.1 to +4.9)	1.28 (1.04 to 1.57)
SHINE Infants of HIV-positive women	No IYCF	6.1	Reference	Reference
	IYCF	6.8	+0.7 (−2.9 to +4.9)	1.12 (0.62 to 2.03)
	No WASH	7.5	Reference	Reference
	WASH	5.6	−1.9 (−10.0 to +6.2)	0.73 (0.40 to 1.33)

WASH, Water, Sanitation, and Hygiene; SHINE, Sanitation Hygiene Infant Nutrition Efficacy; IYCF, infant and young child feeding.

−0.27 (1.03) in Kenya, −0.26 (1.08) in Zimbabwe HIV-unexposed, and −0.55 (1.08) in Zimbabwean HIV-exposed children. Notably, the Nutrition and Nutrition + WASH interventions significantly improved HCZ by 0.16 (0.04–0.27) and 0.11 (0.01–0.20), respectively, in Bangladesh. IYCF also increased HCZ by 0.07 (0.00–0.14) among HIV-unexposed children in Zimbabwe.

None of the WASH interventions had any effect on linear, ponderal, or head growth among any of the study populations.

Outcome: 7-Day Prevalence of Diarrhea
The impact of the randomized interventions on 7-day prevalence of diarrhea (1 and 2 years after interventions, combined in the WASH Benefits trials and at 18 months infant age in the SHINE trial), is presented in Table 3. The prevalence of diarrhea in the control arms was lowest in Bangladesh (5.7%), greater in Zimbabwe (6.1–9.9%), and greatest in Kenya (27.1%).

In WASH Benefits Bangladesh, all the interventions, except water treatment alone, significantly reduced the prevalence of diarrhea by a relative 35–40%. The water treatment intervention reduced diarrhea by a relative 11%, but this difference was not statistically significant. In contrast, none of the interventions reduced diarrhea prevalence in either African site.

Implications

The WASH Benefits and SHINE trials tested the independent and combined effects of an intervention to improve child diet and an intervention to improve household water quality, sanitation, and handwashing behaviors on attained child growth at 18–24 months of age and diarrhea prevalence. The trials delivered hardware (improved latrines, handwashing stations) and commodities (chlorine, soap, and SQ-LNS) at high fidelity. and households took up promoted behaviors at good to high rates creating substantial contrast in indicators of household WASH and infant feeding.

Consistent with decades of complementary feeding research, the IYCF intervention increased linear growth by 0.13–0.26 and reduced stunting by 7–21%. The IYCF intervention also increased weight-for-length Z-score in Bangladesh, among Zimbabwean HIV-unexposed children and in Kenya when given concurrently with WASH.

The sanitation, handwashing, and WASH interventions significantly reduced diarrhea in Bangladesh, but none of the WASH interventions reduced diarrhea in Kenya or Zimbabwe. One important difference between the Bangladesh compared to the African site protocols was the frequency with which behavior change promoters contacted study participants. In Bangladesh, promoters visited 6 times monthly, while in the African sites promoters visited once monthly. On reviewing the literature, virtually all published studies in which point-of-use water chlorination or handwashing promotion reduced diarrhea, high adherence was attained by very frequent contact [23].

The WASH interventions did not improve child linear growth in any of the trials. This lack of effect is most likely because the household-level elementary WASH interventions employed in the trials were not effective enough in reducing enteropathogen exposure to facilitate linear growth. Throughout history, linear growth and child health have improved following substantial socioeconomic development including provision of piped water into homes, sewage systems, and flush toilets. Further evidence emanating from the trials suggest that, although some measures of fecal exposure were reduced (especially well-documented in the WASH Benefits trials), enteropathogen transmission was still

Makasi·Humphrey

substantially higher among children in the WASH arms of these trials compared to children in developed countries. Thus, these trials do not challenge the biological plausibility that excellent WASH services are critical to health, but do challenge the level of WASH interventions typically available to many people in rural areas of low-income countries.

Two consensus documents have called for "Transformative WASH" services that are radically more effective in reducing fecal exposure to be made available to rural low-income populations [23, 24]. "Transformative WASH" may include provision of on-plot, sustained, high-quality water supply (which is articulated in Sustainable Development Goal 6); high community-level sanitation coverage; and new technologies or behavior change modalities. In addition to any of these technologies and interventions, transformative WASH will also require strengthened support for governance systems of financing, operations, monitoring, evaluation, and regulation.

Disclosure Statement

The authors declare no conflicts of interest to disclose.

References

1 UNICEF, WHO, Bank W: Levels and Trends in Child Malnutrition. Joint Child Malnutrition Estimates. New York, United Nations International Children's Fund; Geneva, WHO, Washington, World Bank, 2017.

2 Christian P, Lee SE, Donahue Angel M, et al: Risk of childhood undernutrition related to small-for-gestational age and preterm birth in low- and middle-income countries. Int J Epidemiol 2013; 42:1340–1355.

3 Victora CG, De Onis M, Hallal PC, et al: Worldwide timing of growth faltering: Revisiting implications for interventions. Pediatrics 2010; 125:e473–e480.

4 Prendergast AJ, Humphrey JH: The stunting syndrome in developing countries. Paediatr Int Child Health 2014;34:250–265.

5 Panjwani A, Heidkamp R: Complementary feeding interventions have a small but significant impact on linear and ponderal growth of children in low- and middle-income countries: a systematic review and meta-analysis. J Nutr 2017;147: 2169S–2178S.

6 UNICEF: Strategy for Improved Nutrition of Children and Women in Developing Countries, New York, UNICEF, 1999.

7 Humphrey JH: Child undernutrition, tropical enteropathy, toilets, and handwashing. Lancet 2009;374:1032–1035.

8 Prendergast A, Kelly P: Enteropathies in the developing world: neglected effects on global health. Am J Trop Med Hyg 2012;86:756–763.

9 Sanitation Hygiene Infant Nutrition Efficacy (SHINE) Trial team, Humphrey JH, Jones AD, Manges A, et al: The sanitation hygiene infant nutrition efficacy (SHINE) trial: Rationale, design, and methods. Clin Infect Dis 2015;61(suppl 7):S685–S702.

10 Luby SP, Rahman M, Arnold BF, et al: Effects of water quality, sanitation, handwashing, and nutritional interventions on diarrhoea and child growth in rural Bangladesh: a cluster randomised controlled trial. Lancet Glob Health 2018;6:e302–e315.

11 Null C, Stewart CP, Pickering AJ, et al: Effects of water quality, sanitation, handwashing, and nutritional interventions on diarrhoea and child growth in rural Kenya: a cluster-randomised controlled trial. Lancet Glob Health 2018;6:e316–e329.

12 Humphrey JH, Mbuya MN, Ntozini R, et al: Independent and combined effects of improved water, sanitation, and hygiene, and improved complementary feeding, on child stunting and anaemia in rural Zimbabwe: a cluster-randomised trial. Lancet Glob Health 2019;7:e132–e147.

13 Kwong LH, Ercumen A, Pickering AJ, Unicomb L, Davis J, Luby SP: Hand- and object-mouthing of rural Bangladeshi children 3–18 months old. Int J Environ Res Public Health 2016;13:563.

14 Benjamin-Chung J, Amin N, Ercumen A, et al: A randomized controlled trial to measure spillover effects of a combined water, sanitation, and handwashing intervention in rural Bangladesh. Am J Epidemiol 2018;187:1733–1744.

15 Ercumen A, Pickering AJ, Kwong LH, et al: Animal feces contribute to domestic fecal contamination: evidence from E. coli measured in water, hands, food, flies, and soil in Bangladesh. Environ Sci Technol 2017;51:8725–8734.

16 Ercumen A, Pickering AJ, Kwong LH, et al: Do sanitation improvements reduce fecal contamination of water, hands, food, soil, and flies? Evidence from a cluster-randomized controlled trial in rural Bangladesh. Environ Sci Technol 2018; 52:12089–12097.

17 Pickering AJ, Njenga SM, Steinbaum L, et al: Effects of single and integrated water, sanitation, handwashing, and nutrition interventions on child soil-transmitted helminth and Giardia infections: a cluster-randomized controlled trial in rural Kenya. PLoS Med 2019;16:e1002841.

18 Mbuya MN, Matare CR, Tavengwa NV, et al: Early initiation and exclusivity of breastfeeding in rural Zimbabwe: impact of a breastfeeding intervention delivered by village health workers. Curr Dev Nutr 2019;3:nzy092.

19 Prendergast AJ, Chasekwa B, Evans C, et al: Independent and combined effects of improved water, sanitation, and hygiene, and improved complementary feeding, on stunting and anaemia among HIV-exposed children in rural Zimbabwe: a cluster-randomised controlled trial. Lancet Child Adolesc Health 2019;3:77–90.

20 Caulfield LE, Huffman SL, Piwoz EG: Interventions to improve intake of complementary foods by infants 6 to 12 months of age in developing countries: impact on growth and on the prevalence of malnutrition and potential contribution to child survival. Food and Nutrition Bulletin 1999;20:183–200.

21 Dewey KG, Adu-Afarwuah S: Systematic review of the efficacy and effectiveness of complementary feeding interventions in developing countries. Matern Child Nutr 2008;4(suppl 1):24–85.

22 Scharf RJ, Rogawski ET, Murray-Kolb LE, et al: Early childhood growth and cognitive outcomes: Findings from the MAL-ED study. Matern Child Nutr 2018;14:e12584.

23 Pickering AJ, Null C, Winch PJ, et al: The WASH Benefits and SHINE trials: interpretation of WASH intervention effects on linear growth and diarrhoea. Lancet Glob Health 2019;7:e1139–e1146.

24 Cumming O, Arnold BF, Ban R, et al: The implications of three major new trials for the effect of water, sanitation and hygiene on childhood diarrhea and stunting: a consensus statement. BMC Med 2019;17:173.

Michaelsen KF, Neufeld LM, Prentice AM (eds): Global Landscape of Nutrition Challenges in
Infants and Children. Nestlé Nutr Inst Workshop Ser, vol 93, pp 167–171, (DOI: 10.1159/000504108)
Nestlé Nutrition Institute, Switzerland/S. Karger AG., Basel, © 2020

Summary of Environmental Impacts on Nutrition

Children will achieve their full potential if properly nourished in all meanings of the term, emotionally, educationally, and, of course, nutritionally. But the last of these cannot succeed in isolation from the others. A deeper realization of this truism has fostered the concept of "nutrition-sensitive" factors to complement "nutrition-specific" factors, and it is now abundantly clear that even the best nutrition cannot succeed alone. The manner by which living in an impoverished environment can constrain a child's growth and development is the topic of this session; spanning the parental and fetal epigenome, the effects of the gut microbiome, and the interplay between WASH factors and the so-called environmental enteric disease (EED) that is widely viewed as on the causal pathway of much of the growth failure endemic to low- and middle-income countries (LMICs).

Andrew Prentice set the scene by noting the close interplay between stunting and its associated adverse outcomes for children, ranging from increased risk of death to an association with low (and often deteriorating) head circumference that is assumed to have an impact on their cognitive development [1]. The timing of the growth deficits provides clues as to the nature of the insults. Stunted children are born small, implicating maternal constraints that may combine the effects of an "adapted" epigenome (see article by Silver summarized below [2]) and a poor diet leading up to, and during, pregnancy. Then, compared to the WHO reference values, most children in impoverished environments show a precipitate post-natal drop-off in growth for the first 2 years of life. Thereafter, they stabilize or even start to recover slightly.

While acknowledging that poor diets with low dietary diversity are a major driver of growth failure in young LMIC children, Prentice's chapter emphasizes the other constraints and the physiological mechanisms through which these effects are mediated. Every parent knows that overt infections have a clear effect on appetite and may impair growth. If the child has access to high-quality and sufficient foods during convalescence, growth will recover rapidly; in conditions of poverty, the deficit might persist. Far less appreciated are the likely effects of nonclinical infections. In rural Gambia, for instance, the majority of children turn sero-positive to cytomegalovirus (CMV), Epstein-Barr virus, *Helicobacter pylori*, and, prior to immunization, to hepatitis B virus by their second year of life. Yet, these "silent" infections are never diagnosed by a physician and recorded in their clinic records. Presumably, there is a metabolic cost to fighting these infections, and suppression of the growth axis may be induced to spare energy and nutrients to meet the costs.

Environmental toxins may also impair growth, and, among these, aflatoxin is likely the most prevalent and has been best studied. Prentice summarizes the evidence that aflatoxin contamination of nuts and grains impairs growth possibly through a direct effect on hepatic insulin-like growth factor 1 (IGF1) production [1].

The third category of nonnutritional factors restraining healthy growth in children relates to the very poor hygiene usually associated with living in poverty. Current belief is that this is primarily mediated by a persistent gut damage usually now termed environmental enteric disease (EED). EED is presumed to be caused by the high pathogen and allergen load encountered by young children and at a time when their immune systems have not yet developed their later resilience. EED features cropped villi, crypt hyperplasia, loss of tight junctions, and a chronic, nonresolving inflammatory infiltrate of the gut lining; features that lead to malabsorption and excess utilization of precious nutritional resource.

The final environment-related factor that limits the uptake and utilization of nutrients is inflammation. Using the example of iron, Prentice shows how even very low-grade inflammation causes a hepcidin-mediated blockade of iron absorption and is therefore a critical determinant of anemia.

Ruairi Robertson addresses the possibility that child malnutrition is at least in part caused by a disordered gut microbiome [3]. He first distinguishes the known and important negative effects of enteropathogens from the possible effects – both positive and negative – of commensal organisms. He summarizes the critical role that the gut microbiome plays in maintaining the integrity of the intestinal barrier, in promoting nutrient absorption and metabolic homeostasis, and in modulating immune maturity in the early stages of life.

The early microbiome is influenced by mode of delivery at birth and by exposure to antibiotics and very likely by in utero influences. Breastfed babies have a relatively restricted microbiome dominated by *Bifidobacteria* that utilizing human-milk oligosaccharides. Weaning triggers an expansion in species diversity with abilities to break down complex carbohydrates from the diet.

Robertson then describes new theories and observations regarding *"the microbiome of stunting"* including the suggestion that there is a decompartmentalization in the microbiome with organisms normally restricted to the upper gut colonizing the lower gut and possibly eliciting the chronic inflammation described above. The reverse theory of bacterial overgrowth in the upper gut has been posited for many years to be part of the malnutrition syndrome. He also summarizes theories about *"the microbiome of wasting"* and describes among others the well-known studies from the Gordon lab in which transfer of the "malnourished" microbiome from Malawian twins discordant for malnutrition into germ-free mice was able to recapitulate the malnutrition when the mice were fed a Malawian diet.

There is good evidence that some of the effects of poor diet in inducing growth failure may, in part, be mediated through the gut microbiome. The effects of vitamin A and of nutrients critical to methylation pathways (e.g., choline and folate) are described together with the role of the gut in modulating essential amino acid status. The growing awareness of such effects may aid in the development of "microbiota-directed foods" to specifically target the impaired microbiome in childhood undernutrition.

Finally, Robertson summarizes the current evidence on the potential of various methods of modulating the microbiome to improve child growth, antibiotics, pre- and probiotics, legumes, and fecal microbiome transplantation. While there have been numerous disappointments, the potential scope for such interventions remains encouraging given the pivotal role of the microbiome in directing health.

In a change of tack, Matt Silver described the current state of knowledge regarding the role of epigenetics as a possible modulator of child growth and development [2]. A baby's epigenome, that regulates gene expression, is established in the very early embryo, and these processes are known to be sensitive to the mother's nutritional state; hence, there is every reason to believe that such processes could influence growth. Indeed, there is a thesis that an embryo conceived into a nutrient-poor environment may undergo adaptations that downregulate growth in anticipation of a frugal diet in later life.

Silver sets out the additional possibilities that the echoes of malnutrition in prior generations could limit growth in either an intergenerational or a transgenerational manner; a distinction that is clearly described in his chapter. While entirely plausible, Silver cautions as to how difficult it is to obtain conclusive proof of such processes in humans.

In describing his group's seminal studies on the effects of seasonality in rural Gambia on the establishment of the epigenome in the very early embryo, Silver summarizes evidence that certain genomic regions may have evolved to sense the nutritional environment, record the information on the epigenome, and use this to adapt the fetus to be best aligned to the anticipated future nutritional supply. Such alignment would be beneficial if the environment stayed relatively constant but could be maladaptive if conditions changed. This match-mismatch scenario is posited as a possible mechanism underlying the developmental origins of health and disease.

The final chapter by Jean Humphrey summarizes the results from the recent WASH intervention trials [4]. These large, and excellently conducted, cluster-randomized trials in Bangladesh and Kenya (WASH Benefits) and Zimbabwe (SHINE) studied the effects of interventions aimed at improving water, sanitation, and hygiene (WASH) and of nutrition in the form of improved infant and young child feeding (IYCF) and in various combinations.

The results have been salutary. The IYCF interventions were beneficial, but to a limited extent only with a maximum benefit of about a quarter of one standard deviation for height Z-score; a value in line with other meta-analyses of IYCF interventions in the first 1000 days. The WASH interventions in contrast showed absolutely no benefit on growth despite being implemented with a high level of fidelity and uptake. The salutary element of these trials is that we can safely conclude that interventions based, as these were, on the tenet that they must be cheap in order to be scalable will not work. The WASH Benefits and SHINE trials were conducted so well, and across different LMIC settings, so there will be no need to waste resources on future similar trials. A new approach is needed. Prentice's chapter summarized a natural experiment from which it can be concluded that there is likely a very high WASH threshold that must be reached before child growth will normalize. This is in line with where the field is now moving as policy makers consider what is being termed "Transformative WASH."

Taken together, the papers in this session emphasize how important it is to integrate nutrition interventions with radical improvements in living conditions in order to eliminate malnutrition. The epigenetic insights offer a counsel of patience by suggesting that it may take several generations to move stunted populations in line with the healthy stature of high-income countries and that trying to rush the transformation may induce additional developmental origins of health and disease-related problems of later-life chronic diseases.

Andrew M. Prentice

References

1 Prentice AM: Environmental and Physiological Barriers to Child Growth and Development. In: Michaelsen KF, Neufeld LM, Prentice AM (eds): Global Landscape of Nutrition Challenges in Infants and Children. Nestlé Nutr Inst Workshop Ser. Basel, Karger, 2020, vol 93, pp 125–131.

2 Silver MJ: Intergenerational Influences on Child Development: An Epigenetic Perspective. In: Michaelsen KF, Neufeld LM, Prentice AM (eds): Global Landscape of Nutrition Challenges in Infants and Children. Nestlé Nutr Inst Workshop Ser. Basel, Karger, 2020, vol 93, pp 145–151.

3 Robertson R: The Gut Microbiome in Child Malnutrition. In: Michaelsen KF, Neufeld LM, Prentice AM (eds): Global Landscape of Nutrition Challenges in Infants and Children. Nestlé Nutr Inst Workshop Ser. Basel, Karger, 2020, vol 93, pp 133–143.

4 Makasi R, Humphrey JH: Summarizing the child growth and diarrhoea findings of the WASH Benefits and SHINE trials. In: Michaelsen KF, Neufeld LM, Prentice AM (eds): Global Landscape of Nutrition Challenges in Infants and Children. Nestlé Nutr Inst Workshop Ser. Basel, Karger, 2020, vol 93, pp 153–166.

Subject Index

A&T, *see* Alive and Thrive
ACE, *see* Angiotensin-converting enzyme
Aflatoxin, growth impact 128, 129
Alive and Thrive (A&T) 26–30
Allergy, cow's milk allergy and linear
    growth 81
Amino acids
    composition in plant foods 117
    plants versus meat 114
    ready-to-use supplementary food
        source 114–116
Anemia, *see also* Iron; Vitamin B12
    etiology 8–10, 52, 53
    intervention guidelines 53
Angiotensin-converting enzyme
    (ACE) 138
Antibiotics, growth impact 139

BCTs, *see* Behavior change techniques
Behavior change techniques (BCTs) 27–29
Breastfeeding
    guideline adherence 17–19
    importance 68
    micronutrient concentrations in milk
        adequacy 69, 70
        deficiency risks 70, 71
        measurement
            importance 68
            techniques 71–73
        reference value establishment 74, 75
        supplementation impact 73, 74

CARE 28, 30
CMV, *see* Cytomegalovirus

Complementary feeding, guideline
    adherence 19, 20
Corn-soya blend (CSB) 113
Cow's milk
    adult stature and health outcomes 84,
        85
    age of puberty impact 82, 83
    growth components 85
    high intake negative effects 85, 86
    insulin-like growth factor-I
        response 83, 84
    linear growth outcomes
        allergy impact 81
        intervention studies 80
        observational studies 79, 80
        overview 78
    obesity studies 81, 82
    ready-to-use supplementary food
        proteins 114–116
    recommendations 86
CSB, *see* Corn-soya blend
Cytomegalovirus (CMV) 127, 168

Dairy, *see* Cow's milk
Diarrhea, WASH intervention
    studies 163, 164
Diarrhea, iron intervention 58, 59
DNA methylation, *see* Epigenetics

EED, *see* Environmental enteric disease
Environmental enteric disease
    (EED) 127, 128, 134, 154, 167, 168
Epigenetics, nutritional
    programming 145–150

Epstein-Barr virus 127, 168

FCDB, *see* Food composition tables and databases
Fecal microbiome transplantation (FMT) 140
Ferritin, iron status biomarker 54
FMT, *see* Fecal microbiome transplantation
Folate
  folic acid supplementation versus natural folates 93
  vitamin B12 action comparison 93
Food composition tables and databases (FCDB)
  data sources 40, 41
  global availability 44–46
  global initiatives 46, 47
  limitations for micronutrient intake estimation
    food composition variability 41–43
    quality of tables and databases 43, 44
  overview 40
  prospects 47, 48
Fortification
  food-based strategies 33–35
  micronutrient powder 30–33
FUT 96, 97

Gut microbiome
  colonization 135
  dietary insufficiency and undernutrition impact 138, 139
  environmental enteric disease 134, 136
  malnutrition impact 134
  stunting studies 136, 137, 169
  targeting in malnutrition
    antibiotics 139
    fecal microbiome transplantation 140
    legumes 140
    probiotics 139, 140
  wasting studies 137, 138

Helicobacter pylori 127, 168
Hepatitis B 127, 168

Hepcidin, iron status biomarker 54, 55
HFP, *see* Homestead food production
HIV, *see* Human immunodeficiency virus
Homestead food production (HFP), Helen Keller International program 34
Human immunodeficiency virus (HIV) 127

IGF-I, *see* Insulin-like growth factor-I
Infant and young child feeding (IYCF), guidelines
  adherence
    breastfeeding 17–19
    caregiver feeding styles 20, 21
    complementary feeding 19, 20
    prospects for study 21, 22
  assessment 17
  global recommendations 16, 17
Infection, growth impact
  environmental enteric disease 127, 128
  subclinical infection 126, 127
Inflammation, growth impact of chronic low-grade inflammation 129, 130
INFOODS, *see* International Network of Food Data Systems
Insulin-like growth factor-I (IGF-I)
  aflatoxin effects 129
  cow's milk response 83, 84
International Network of Food Data Systems (INFOODS) 46, 47
Iodine
  breast milk composition 70
  vegan diet 107
Iron, *see also* Anemia
  breast milk composition 69
  deficiency prevalence 54, 55
  toxicity 60
  universal intervention benefits
    anemia improvement 56
    cognitive development 56, 57
    diarrhea 58, 59
    growth 57
    malaria 57, 58
    overview 55
    respiratory tract infection 59, 60
  vegan diet 107

IYCF, *see* Infant and young child feeding

Jeevan-Jyothi 30, 31

Legumes, gut microbiome effects 139, 140

Malaria, iron intervention 57, 58
Malnutrition, *see also* Obesity; Stunting
    etiology 6–11
    global burden 2–5, 134
    progress against 5, 6
    treatment
        moderate acute malnutrition 113,
          116–118
        severe acute malnutrition 112–115
Microbiota, *see* Gut microbiome
Micronutrient powder (MNP)
    Jeevan-Jyothi project 30, 31
    Pushtikona project 31–33
Milk, *see* Breastfeeding; Cow's milk
MNP, *see* Micronutrient powder

Obesity
    cow's milk studies 81, 82
    etiology 10, 11

Probiotics 139, 140
Pushtikona 31–33

Ready-to-use supplementary food
    (RUTF) 113–117
Respiratory tract infection, iron
    intervention 59, 60
RUTF, *see* Ready-to-use supplementary
    food

Sanitation Hygiene Infant Nutrition
    Efficacy (SHINE) 155–163, 170
SBCC, *see* Social sand behavior change
    communication
SHINE, *see* Sanitation Hygiene Infant
    Nutrition Efficacy
Social sand behavior change
    communication (SBCC)
    A&T 26–30
    overview of nutrition
        interventions 26–28

Stunting
    epidemiology 154
    etiology 8
    gut microbiome studies 136, 137, 169

TCN1 96
TCN II 97
Transferrin receptor, iron status
    biomarker 54, 55

Vegan diet
    definitions 104, 105
    nutrient coverage 106–108
    recommendations 108, 109
Vitamin B6, breast milk composition 73
Vitamin B12
    absorption and transport 95–97
    breast milk composition 70, 72, 73
    folate action comparison 93
    intervention studies in India 94–101
    pernicious anemia versus nutrient
        deficiency 92, 93
    supplementation in laction 73, 74
    synthesis 91, 92
    vegan diet 108, 122
Vitamin D
    breast milk composition 69
    vegan diet 107

WASH, *see* Water, sanitation, and hygiene
Wasting, gut microbiome studies 137, 138
Water, sanitation, and hygiene (WASH)
    environmental enteric disease 127, 128
    growth outcome trials
        diarrhea prevalence 163, 164
        implications 164, 165
        Sanitation Hygiene Infant Nutrition
          Efficacy 155–163
        WASH Benefits Bangladesh 155–
          163, 170
        WASH Benefits Kenya 155–163, 170
    thresholds to normalize child
        growth 130

Zinc
    breast milk composition 69
    vegan diet 107